KINFLIX

FORMATIONS: ADOPTION, KINSHIP, AND CULTURE

Emily Hipchen and John McLeod, Series Editors

KINFLIX

ADOPTION AND ASSISTED REPRODUCTIVE TECHNOLOGIES IN FILM

Marina Fedosik

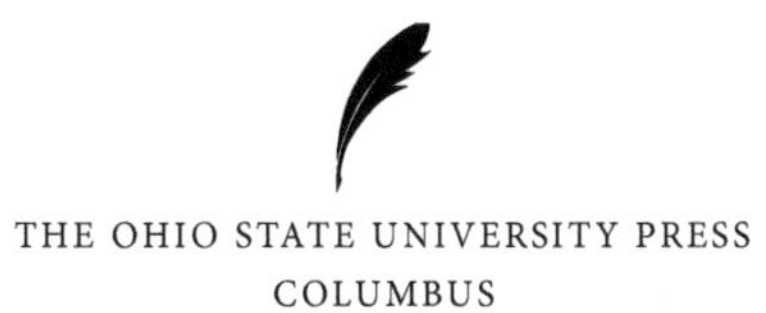

THE OHIO STATE UNIVERSITY PRESS
COLUMBUS

Published by The Ohio State University Press.

Library of Congress Cataloging-in-Publication Data

Names: Fedosik, Marina, author

Title: Kinflix : adoption and assisted reproductive technologies in film / Marina Fedosik.

Other titles: Formations: adoption, kinship, and culture

Description: Columbus : The Ohio State University Press, [2025] | Series: Formations: adoption, kinship, and culture | Includes bibliographical references and index. | Summary: "Analyzes cinematic representations of adoption and technologically assisted reproduction to identify the intersecting paradigms through which Western cultures understand these ways of making families"—Provided by publisher.

Identifiers: LCCN 2025028397 | ISBN 9780814215197 hardback | ISBN 081421519X hardback | ISBN 9780814284476 ebook | ISBN 0814284477 ebook

Subjects: LCSH: Adoption in motion pictures | Human reproductive technology in motion pictures | Reproductive technology | Motion pictures, American—20th century—History and criticism | Motion pictures, American—21st century—History and criticism

Classification: LCC PN1995.9.A28 F43 2025

LC record available at https://lccn.loc.gov/2025028397

Other identifiers: ISBN 9780814259634 (paperback) | ISBN 0814259634 (paperback)

Cover design by Charles Brock
Text design by Juliet Williams
Type set in Adobe Minion Pro

♾ The paper used in this publication meets the minimum requirements of the American National Standard for Information Sciences—Permanence of Paper for Printed Library Materials. ANSI Z39.48-1992.

CONTENTS

ILLUSTRATIONS

INTRODUCTION

Adoption and Other Forms of Post-Heterocoital Reproduction

> I believe that there will be no racial or sexual peace, no livable nature, until we learn to reproduce humanity through something more and less than kinship.
>
> —Donna Haraway, "Universal Donors" (366)

In Steven Spielberg's *A.I. Artificial Intelligence* (2001), Monica, a human adoptive mother of a robot boy, David, takes her mecha (mechanical) son into the woods after several months of living together. She leaves him there because it is inconceivable for her to have him as part of her family, and yet she does not want to return David to the manufacturer because he will be destroyed. Monica cannot bring herself to "kill" David because he looks "so real," "just like a child," and he evokes profound empathy in humans. But in response to David's pleas not to leave him alone, she shouts as she runs away, "You are not real!" With these words, Monica denies David's wish to be included in a human family on a footing equal to a human son. She also refuses to consider her feelings for David real. Her decision to abandon him in the woods rests on a conviction that their kinship is fake, deceptive, and therefore can be justifiably terminated. The scene foregrounds David's origin—a manufactured mecha that can only pass as, never be, an orga (organic human)—as the reason for the derealization of this kinship. Monica's feelings elicited by this simulacrum of a human programmed to love his human family are experienced by her as a dangerous delusion that threatens her sanity and the safety of other family members. Unlike an organic body of a human child that originates in the natural heterocoital act of its parents, David's mechanical body is technologically produced, and this difference in origin determines what he "is" and what place he can take within human kinship relationships.

The focus of *A.I.* on robot adoption as a simulacrum of human kinship most obviously invites exploration of anxieties around the place of technology in human life. Such anxieties often manifest themselves as concerns over the difficulty in drawing a distinction between the real and the artificial, and the nonacceptance of techno-human hybridity. Less obvious but more interesting for the purposes of this book are the connections drawn between such anxieties and ideas about human reproduction, origin, and kinship. Beyond understanding David's body as a product of technology, *A.I.* invites looking at adoption itself as a reproductive technology, albeit familiar enough not to register as such in the conventional sense. Robot adoption makes the manipulation of traditional kinship visible by separating biological and social reproduction and profoundly unsettles the biocultural consistency that typically underlies Western kinship practices. In this way, this adoption limit case sets the stage for the tension between the natural and the manufactured that structures cultural discourses about adoption and more recent technologies of assisted reproduction.

More specifically, the film presages the problem of the reproductive difference, a consequence of diverse modes of reproduction that may confer different degrees of humanity on entities whose origins differ from those traditionally recognized as human. David is adopted by Monica and her husband, Henry, as a substitute for the couple's biogenetic son, Martin, who is cryogenically frozen while a cure for his life-threatening disease is being developed. It is important that Monica's decision to abandon David comes after Martin is cured and returns home. While obviously David's ultimate abandonment is motivated by the perceived threat he presents to Martin's well-being and life (he accidentally almost drowns Martin in a swimming pool), Monica's decision to take David to the woods, instead of back to the factory where he would be scrapped like an obsolete machine, suggests that he is perceived as less than human yet more than a robot, a child substitute. In this way, the film overlays the hierarchy of "real-ness" along the human-machine continuum onto the distinctions between "real" / "not real" child of one's own. While *A.I.* is dealing with a limit case of human adoption of a robot, its representational logic suggests possible cultural consequences for kinship facilitated through reproductive technologies and practices in which the certainty about traditional human origin may be diluted and kinship is not always or not firmly grounded in biogenetic continuity.

The cinematic narratives analyzed in this book represent a range of nontraditional reproductive options, beginning with adoption that troubles the traditional understanding of "real" kinship by creating a configuration with two sets of parents: the biological-heterocoital and the adoptive ones. As a logical extension of this line of inquiry, this book also ventures into narratives of assisted reproduction, both already available and potentially possible, that may disrupt accepted understandings of reproduction and kinship even further. As an anchor point for analysis, this book defines traditional reproductive human origin as *heterocoital,* that is, the result of a heterosexual reproductive act between two genitors of the opposing (binary, male/female) sex. The possibility of producing a child whose origin differs from the heterocoital creates further cultural anxieties around assisted reproduction technologies (ARTs) because they may introduce into the process a number of genitors different from the conventional heterosexual two. *Kinflix* concerns itself with such anxieties and examines representations of non-heterocoital reproduction in narrative cinema to understand the ways in which cultural ideas about human reproduction and kinship respond to reproductive technologies as they shape our values, social lives, and affective scripts we live by. The analysis of nontraditional reproduction in narrative Western cinema ultimately shows that even in the absence of the heterocoital act, reproductive capacity, and the heterosexuality traditionally understood as the cultural bedrock of reproduction, patriarchy-inflected Western cultures aim to preserve heterocoital logic of kinship as they come to terms with technological advances in human reproduction.

The selection of films does not follow any specific chronology, even though most of them were made in the second half of the twentieth and the beginning of the twenty-first centuries when the discussion of adoption and assisted reproduction has become more culturally prominent. The selection of films is an attempt to pull together a corpus of texts that includes well-known films that have produced a noticeable cultural response together with lesser-known ones and limit cases that show something significant about our imaginaries of nontraditional reproduction. These categories offer a gamut of conventional cultural approaches to nontraditional reproduction as well as ways to challenge the status quo.

While much attention is paid to the specifics of representations of adoption and ART in visual texts, the end goal of the book is to uncover the overarching logic of cultural thinking about human biological and social reproduction, including conceptual shifts in accepted ideas as well as cultural resistances to such changes. This tug-of-war, staged in nontraditional reproduction narratives, signals the need to meet ongoing technological changes with new ways of thinking about human identity, kinship, and resultant social formations. The chapters of the book examine the logic of nontraditional reproduction representations in different genres of cinema in order to uncover possible reasons for insistence on heterocoital origin as a matter of humanity.

By extending thinking into the territory where a child's heterocoital origin is unknown, uncertain, or does not exist and therefore cannot be called upon to secure personhood and belonging as a matter of culturally established and institutionalized heterocoital frameworks, narratives of nontraditional reproduction push us to consider consequences of non-heterocoital reproductive and kinship practices for our social life and especially their stakes for entities whose universally recognized human origin is in question.

Some of such consequences have already been foreshadowed in critical adoption studies (CAS)—a field that critically examines ideas about origins, kinship, family, identity, and belonging that are often taken for granted.[1] For example, cultural insistence on heterocoital origin as a condition for a recognizable social identity is revealed by an essential adoption paradox. The cultural demand to develop and maintain an adoptive kinship bond indistinguishable from biogenetic affiliation is persistently coupled with this bond's constant "derealization" (Butler 114) by imagining it as just like the real one. Adoption revealed early the presence of such cultural imperatives through the existence of adoption-specific double binds. Time and time again, the cultural distinction between adoptive and "real"—in other words, heterocoital—kinship compels adoption participants to negotiate paradoxes of identity and belonging that originate from this dichotomy. For example, Barbara Melosh observes that, typically, in Western cultures the adoptive family has to appear "as if begotten," and yet it is perpetually measured against the biological model it can never fully replicate (2009, 104). Sally Sales invokes a similar double bind when she explains that the adoptee's individualization and personhood depend on simultaneous identification and differentiation from the "original [biological] kin" (6). Sales demonstrates that the Western, middle-class cultural process of individuation depends on biogenetic origin knowledge, and so the adopted child's origin is always constitutive to the adoptive family and adoptee's selfhood. This identity-belonging paradigm persists whether the cultural imperative is to hide and repress the biogenetic origin of the child or to acknowledge and cultivate it.

What Sales names the "dual and contradictory message at the centre of adoption practices" (8) reveals a tension between cultural ideas about kinship. On the one hand, adoption is celebrated for its transcendence of biogenetic relatedness in kinship formation, while on the other hand, it still must contend with cultural insistence on heterocoital origin knowledge as a universal condition for human personhood. Whether it is a closed or open adoption,

1. "Critical" in this context does not mean criticizing adoption or discussing its abolition, although these perspectives are examined in CAS scholarship.

Sales found, the family is expected to "provide the child with a new foundation, but simultaneously sustain the old foundation of the [biological] family origin" (8). Such sustaining can look like acknowledgment of a child's adopted status, curating narratives of a child's transfer between parents, celebrating "gotcha" days, support for the adoptees' engagement with their birth culture and families, et cetera. Adoptees may feel willing or compelled to come to terms with such insistence through the right-to-know movements and return trips. The perpetually negotiable discourse of the best interest of the child aims to reconcile children's belonging with their biological parents and their transfer to the adoptive family. The duality serves to simultaneously ensure adoptive family unity and to legitimate the adoptee's personhood in a culture that relies on the knowledge of heterocoital origin as the universal basis of identity and belonging.

The need to manage the disruptive effect of such duality is seen in cultural production that aims to contain its effects on ideas about reproduction and human identity. For example, in response to cultural expectations for proper identity formation that demand heterocoital origin knowledge, search and reunion adoption narratives, one of the most popular genres of adoption representation, have emerged.[2] They come to terms with the "bio-genealogical imperative" (Latchford 4) by presenting an adoptee's search for and a possible reunion with a biological family as a pivotal step in personhood development. The "family romance" fantasy,[3] specifically, is often resolved by a reaffirmation of the adopted person's belonging with the adoptive family after the adoptee completes their heterocoital origin search. The reaffirmation can be represented as the adoptee calling the adoptive parents "mom and dad," openly stating their love for the adoptive family, continuing to live at the adoption location, and so on. Sometimes, search narratives include birth parents' acknowledgment of the adoptive family's primacy in the adoptee's life. While not every adopted person searches, not every one chooses the adoptive family as a site of primary emotional investment, and not every one stays in the adoptive country after the search, narratives that gain visibility and cultural weight are the ones that feature an adopted person reinstating kinship ties with the adoptive family after being healed by a recovery of their heterocoital origin. Katarina Wegar cites George Gerbner's study, which has shown that

2. See Melosh (2002); Cartwright; Homans (2006); Novy; Fedosik (2009b), among others, for discussions of search and reunion narratives.

3. The family romance is a psychological complex described by Sigmund Freud in his essay "The Family Romances" (1909). It is a defense mechanism a child may develop against its parents' inability to satisfy the child's needs. It is expressed as the child's fantasy of being adopted, accompanied by idealization of their imaginary "real" parents.

popular culture portrayals of adoption that focused on the adopted person's search for their heterocoital parents exceeded the actual ratio of such searches by up to eighteen times and that most media search narratives resolved in the reconfirmed unity of adoptive family, even though the search for heterocoital origin is at the center of the search plot (110). Wegar concludes that "the rise of the search narrative as the most popular type of adoption story in American mass media . . . is not coincidental but mirrors a contemporary anxiety over the fate of the family and the strength of kinship bonds" (119).[4]

This anxiety is managed through a peculiar dialectic that does not resolve in an erasure or a synthesis of the reproductive configuration duality characteristic of adoption. The cultural work search narratives do is more complex than establishing the biological family as the adoptee's site of origin and primal belonging. The main ethical thrust of the search narrative—to confirm the importance of the biogenetic bond between the parent and the child—is persistently coupled with a reaffirmation of the adoptive family (a.k.a. culturally constructed kinship) as a good enough imitation of the biogenetic family bonds. These negotiations stem from the cultural assumptions that to be a human person, one needs to know their heterocoital origin, and that one's heterocoital origin is synonymous with one's nuclear family that raises them. Trying to come to terms with this assumption, the existent literature on adoption, both scholarly and nonacademic, has attempted to bridge or transcend such duality, often by adjusting the articulation of the adoptee's origin. For example, adoptees may claim belonging to both birth and adoptive families and cultures, yet not fully to any of them.[5] Some adoptees invent a new ontological category (e.g., the transnational adoptee) grounded in difference from conventional personhoods defined by bloodlines or by national or racial belonging. And some discourses locate the "nature" of the adopted child (as per the Hague Convention) in the process of transition from one place and parent to another.[6] But, to reapply an observation by Margaret Homans, "positions such as those . . . remain for the most part locked in the binary opposition" between

4. In analyzing the sealed records movement, Wegar argues that cultural ideology that stresses the importance of biogenetic bonds compels the adoptees and birth parents to search and demand openness in adoption. She argues against understanding the need to know as an essentialist and universal need, in favor of thinking of this need as induced by culture. Since "this society knowledge about genetic heritage is generally regarded and experienced as an important part of a person's identity, perhaps even as an archetypal yearning," she claims that "it is both cruel and unreasonable to expect adoptees and their biological parents to feel otherwise" (137, 136–37). Also see the scholarship of Kimberly Leighton on this issue.

5. See search and reunion memoirs by Trenka; Robinson, among many others.

6. Barbara Yngvesson, ctd. in Jerng (2008). In this latter method, the insistence on knowing the origin and thus the distinction between biological versus adopted is still preserved, even though the primacy of one site of belonging over the other is unsettled.

biogenetic origin and adoptive kinship (2013, 17). In this dualistic hierarchy, the biogenetic is typically valued above the adoptive.

Such effects of adoption have presaged cultural anxieties around more technologically advanced ways of human (re)production and affiliation that push the boundaries of what is considered "real" personhood and kinship even further. In *The Adoption and Donor Conception Factbook,* Lori Carangelo cites the 2010 survey done for the Institute for American Values by Karen Clark, Norval Glenn, and Elizabeth Marquardt on "how Donor Offspring really fare and feel" (129). Among other things, the survey compares adopted and donor-conceived individuals and reports that "on average, young adults conceived through sperm donation are hurting more, are more confused and feel more isolated from their families than those who were *either adopted or raised by their biological families*" (130). Carangelo acknowledges criticisms of the survey's "questionable methodology" (130), but the ethos of the survey is echoed by other sources collected in the *Factbook,* both popular reports and scholarly studies, and this consistency reflects broader cultural attitudes to nontraditional ways of reproduction and family making. Among the concerns donor-conceived individuals have, the survey mentions feeling "confused about who is a member of their family and who is not," "fear [of] being attracted to or having sexual relations" with someone genetically related, concerns about knowing the truth of their origin, fear that their attempts to search for their biogenetic parent may hurt feelings of the parents that are raising them (131), and concern over the money that was involved in their conception process (132). Individuals raised by single mothers wondered about their biological father more often than children raised by heterosexual or same-sex couples and were more likely to think that the donor was a significant part of "who [they were]" (131). The results of the survey constellate to explain positions like David Velleman's, which was critiqued by Sally Haslanger as reliant on unexamined assumptions that being raised by one's biological parents is morally imperative. Such "bionormativ[e]" reasoning (Haslanger) foregrounds biogenetic, heterocoital origin as the basis of human identity. The pervasiveness and longevity of the cultural ideas these sources reveal are confirmed, for example, by a 2020 survey of donor-conceived (DC) individuals interested in finding out about their origin, which shows that 80 percent of them attempted to make contact with the donor and 74 percent were inclined to refer to them as their biological mother or father.[7] Only 9 percent did not want any relationship with the donor. A 2021 study by Burke and colleagues found that 85 percent of surveyed DC individuals experienced "a shift in their 'sense of

7. See "2022 Survey"; see also Burke et al.

self'" after finding out the truth about their origin. It is interesting that Carangelo's collection of evidence shows that reproductive difference marked by adoption seems more culturally acceptable than assisted reproduction. If it is the "normalcy" of the adoptee's assumed heterocoital origin that confers such preference, ART conception, even though it may be concealed and presented as heterocoital, may produce stronger anxieties due to less easily identifiable conventional (a.k.a. heterocoital) anchors of origin and belonging.

Social challenges presented by non-heterocoital reproduction and kinship expose the dependence of human personhood and belonging on cultural scripts of individuation and filiation that require heterocoital origin knowledge. This way of thinking about kinship, as Judith Butler shows in *Undoing Gender,* is tightly connected to the project of social reproduction through uninterrupted culture transmission. By analyzing structuralist ideas about culture that can be traced back to Claude Lévi-Strauss's *The Elementary Structures of Kinship,* Butler shows that even though ideas developed in this work have since been "surpassed" (119), they keep informing cultural objections to nonnormative kinship formations because they serve as a platform for imagining the reproduction of culture in toto as biological, heterosexual reproduction. Butler explains that according to a "certain anthropological belief that is shared by many Lacanian followers" (118), "the culture itself requires that a man and a woman produce a child and that the child have this dual point of reference for its own initiation into the symbolic order, where the symbolic order consists of a set of rules that order that order and support our sense of reality and cultural intelligibility" (118). Within such a framework, the "dual point of reference" (118) is necessary because the entrance into the symbolic order and the child's acceptance of heterosexuality as one of its "rules" depends on successful oedipalization[8]—a developmental process in which a child's desire to possess the mother is regulated by the father, who prevents a full union (sexual or not) of the mother and the child.

Butler's ideas suggest that perpetuation of heteronormativity is behind the culturally imperative bionormativity. While there are differences in cultural ideas about adoption and ARTs, they share the belief that continuity of culture is naturally connected to biological, heterosexual reproduction. Butler showcases the importance of this belief when she observes that the child "figures in the debate" around access to adoption and reproductive technology "as a dense site for the transfer and reproduction of culture" (110). According to her, cultural transfer imagined as a consequence of biological reproduction

8. Throughout the book, the term *oedipal* and its derivatives will be applied in analysis as used in the scholarly conversation engaged in each particular moment. Overall, it gestures toward and describes family and identity dynamics theorized in heterocoital nuclear families.

depends on maintaining heterosexuality as a naturalized cultural norm. The bionormative family, tasked with reproducing culture in this way, works to conflate nature and culture in order to reproduce "not the culturally variable formations of human life, but the universal conditions for human intelligibility" (118). In other words, the family grounded in heterosexual (assumed heterocoital) reproduction serves to produce a reality in which gendered reproductive subjects ensure further reproduction of bodies and of the heterocoital symbolic order they live to maintain. Culturally legible identities and forms of belonging emerge against nonnormative subject positions excluded from the "natural" system of human relatedness.

The example of robot adoptee David, more fully analyzed in chapter 4 of this book, shows how devaluation of non-heterocoital origin may be caused by cultural imaginings of an adoptee or an ART-reproduced person as unable to properly complete oedipalization or to resolve the family romance fantasy—two psychic processes considered fundamental to identity development and familial belonging within the heterocoital symbolic order. *A.I.*, as do other narratives considered in this book, reflects and reveals Lacanian underpinnings of the cultural scripts for individuation and belonging that David aims to follow in his quest to become "real," or, in other words, to be recognized as a son of a human family. But David's portrayed failure shows the impossibility of his project within a culture that considers biogenetic heterocoital origin a "universal conditio[n] of human intelligibility" (Butler 118). His non-heterocoital identity, a harbinger of possible human ontologies in which technological and biological can be hard to separate, remains beyond the frame of reference considered by most Western cultures necessary for cultural (self-)recognition as a "human" who deserves inclusion into the system of human relatedness as a legible and legitimate subject. Such cultural failure to account for reproductive difference shows that the more reproductive technologies move away from the imitation of traditional heterocoital reproduction, the more the need for a revision of heterocoital symbolic order becomes apparent.

It may seem logical that the new, wider range of kinship possibilities facilitated by nontraditional reproductive technologies and practices should revise the heterocoital imperative and expand the registry of human identities and forms of belonging. And yet, Western cultures perpetuate conservative adherence to scripts of relatedness and structures of feelings typical of the model of kinship organized around compulsory heterosexuality, oedipalization, and knowledge of heterocoital origin. Some scholars see the potential of nontraditional kinship formations to transcend the "binary opposition between the given and the constructed" and lead us toward "a non-dualistic understanding of nature-culture interaction" (Braidotti 2013, 3). Butler, for instance, sees the "clearly salutary consequences" of adoption and donor insemination, which she imagines as ushering in "the breakdown of the symbolic order" (127). She believes in the potential of the "relations of filiation . . . not based on biology" (126) to redefine kinship by "opening [it] to a set of community ties that are irreducible to family" (127). Such redefinition, in turn, would destabilize the boundaries between categories of otherness (re)produced within kinship structures that are organized around the heterosexual model and biological descent. But Butler herself has noticed in her analysis of gay marriage rights in France that objections to nonheterosexual marriage often increase when the issue of adoption is on the table. And, as we now know, many donor-conceived children demand the right to know their donor's information and even search for their siblings whose origin can be traced back to the same donor.

As Frances Latchford demonstrates in *Steeped in Blood,* a varying degree of injury to the sense of self and belonging may be experienced by the people whose heterocoital and legal origins differ: it may be felt by the adoptees who know that they were adopted but have no way of finding information about their biological parents or by the children brought to life through donor insemination who do not have a father in the traditional sense. Latchford observes that adoptees are "differentiated from biological children," and they are not "equally valued when they do not know or cannot access their biogenealogies" (4). In such cases, though, the origin can still be connected to a man and a woman and thus, albeit narratively, folded back into the heterocoital framework. In fact, the social imperative for the adoptive family to be "just like" the heterocoital family serves to reimagine adoption in terms of heterocoital reproduction, and it demands that the adoptee confirm their heterocoital origin by knowing that they have heterocoital, a.k.a. "birth" parents. But future reproductive technologies may introduce more variables and unknowns destabilizing to human personhood. For instance, the technology of mitochondrial replacement, in which mitochondrial DNA is donated by a "third biological parent,"[9] further destabilizes the connection of biological origins to normative heterosexuality. In-vitro gametogenesis (IVG) "enables solo reproduction" by using a single individual's cells to produce both female and male gametes (Notini et al. 125). Unlike cloning, this reproductive process creates a new, unique individual who can have just one biological parent. In other cases, as in mitochondrial donation or gamete donation combined with surrogacy, the number of participants biologically involved in the process of reproduction can expand beyond the culturally acceptable heterocoital

9. The scientific community is wary of such terminology, but it has been used in the popular media reports on mitochondrial donation, which is indicative of the cultural response to such innovations.

dyad. Such non-heterocoital configurations elicit cultural resistance expressed as the need to renaturalize some reproductive practices and to stigmatize or ban the ones that are obvious departures from the heterocoital framework. For instance, IVG is typically considered acceptable for opposite-sex couples because it is perceived as therapeutic in cases of infertility. In this context, it is seen as restoring a couple's natural capacity for heterosexual reproduction. But in cases of same-sex and solo reproduction, IVG is generally perceived as suspect by the larger culture because it would be "provided for social [as opposed to 'natural'] reasons" (Notini et al. 126).

The analysis of cinematic texts in this book shows that all the new developments notwithstanding, so far, the cultural significance of the heterocoital kinship model does not seem to be significantly reduced by the advent of ARTs, and even "radical" kinship formations through various reproductive technologies demand the "rooting of identity in an originary biological heritage" that "appears to be an abiding practice at the heart of western kinship" (Sales 8). The cultural primacy of the heterocoital family is reinscribed by the use of the heterocoital family as a "metaphor[ ] we live by" (Lakoff and Johnson 1) with the power to structure all kinds of kinship according to its logic.

Kinflix explores the work of this metaphor by examining popular representations of adoption and ARTs in film as both indicative and formative of cultural ideas and scripts that give shape to Western adoption and other non-heterocoital kinship-building and identity formation practices. The book's focus on film as the domain of analysis is prompted by the growing importance of this medium as a source of cultural literacy. Film and TV, as representational media, have become as influential and formative of contemporary subjectivities as novels were for the emerging middle class in the nineteenth century.[10] Extending this argument to cinematic representations more broadly, we can see that in the increasingly visual, rather than print, culture, the cinematic image has become the vehicle that serves to (re)produce cultural knowledge about adoption and ARTs. While in opinion polls respondents have consistently named family, friends, and the news as their top two sources for information about adoption, films are still cited as a source of such information.[11] The difference and significance of films as sources is in the kind of information they provide. While the news and word of mouth may provide immediate, specific, operational information, films

10. As Greg Metcalf writes in *The DVD Novel*, "Watching shows has become like reading a novel" (x).

11. In the survey by Evan B. Donaldson Adoption Institute, 6 percent of respondents named films as sources of information about adoption, and in a survey by Dave Thomas Foundation for Adoption, the number was 10 percent.

provide culturally stabilized narratives about reproduction characteristic of a specific time. Adoption scholars generally consider films as sources for the public imaginings of what adoption is. For instance, Christine Ward Gailey says that "movies play an important role in providing metaphors and images that people use in thinking about a range of social issues," including adoption (71). Gailey further points out that even if the viewers may take different affective stances to what they see, they are still shaped by the ideas conveyed from the screen. In her study, she observed adopters' and adoptees' reactions to cinematic representations of adoption ranging "from acceptance to skepticism to rejection," but the impact of cinematic portrayals of adoption on personal understanding of adoption was universal (71). Marianne Novy, too, points out that even the adoption participants' experiences of adoption can be shaped and informed by narratives circulating in the culture (1). Susan Bordo claims that cinematic representations are "what we have to inform our public 'imaginary' about adoption" (323). And Sandra Patton in *Birth Marks* notices that cultural cinematic production can influence public policymaking because "legislative agendas do not exist in isolation from popular culture and public opinion" but, rather, "draw on broader social stories about race and identity, gender and family, class and work, that are widely available in popular culture" (132–33).[12] In turn, public policy can be acculturated through popular culture. For example, transracial adoption legislation of the early 1990s caused "a wave of television talk shows, made-for-television movies, and cinematic films . . . about adoption, foster care, and the relative 'fitness' or otherwise of poor and middle-class mothers" (Patton 132). Nontraditional reproduction films recurrently engage viewers with narratives that reaffirm the primacy of heterocoital family and origin by casting non-heterocoital kinship as reproductive difference. According to Heather Jacobson (2014), representations of adoption in the media have been criticized for "cast[ing] adoption as clearly outside the norm"[13] and focusing on "problems thought to besiege 'nontraditional' families" (655). In the process of solidifying heterocoital family and origin as anchors for human identity and personhood, "adoption [is represented as] Other in a culture and kinship system organized by biological reproduction" (Melosh 2004, 218). Thus, we can understand the work of the film as contouring cultural values that are acceptable to the larger culture.[14] Given

12. For additional analysis of popular culture representations of adoption in film, see vol. 9, no. 2 (2021) of *Adoption and Culture* journal.

13. For similar critiques, also see Kline et al. (2006, 2009); Pertman.

14. Public perception of films as didactic can be seen, for example, in a 1995 survey by *The Los Angeles Times* that found that 77 percent of respondents valued "movies that reflect public values, even if it means sacrificing creativity."

that, literacy in reading visual narratives becomes an important part of one's cultural intelligence.

While the overarching structuring methodology that holds the book together aims at deciphering the ways in which adoption and ARTs are "translated" in cinematic representations into heterocoital frameworks, genre-specific structuring of chapters has its specific reasons. By the virtue of its formalized aesthetic, genre cinema crystallizes cultural scripts for and attitudes to different forms of kinship and genealogical identities. In other words, film genres can be analyzed as modes that channel our processing of experiences into genre-specific affective scripts that establish our emotional and moral stances toward certain kinds of reproduction, belonging, and identities. These scripts are widely consumed by the public through the medium that deeply engages the audience's emotional responses and has a great power to inform the audience's cultural and affective stances toward their lived experience. Such universalization and standardization of our responses is akin to an ideology that serves to maintain a social order. The order is underpinned by shared affective experiences that pull individuals' feelings toward socially appropriate affective stances, which, in turn, create attraction and aversion toward certain kinds of experiences and cultural formations.

That said, analysis in this book resists simple ideological readings of film genres. It observes, instead, how cinematic narratives of non-heterocoital kinship and reproduction navigate the tension between the natural and the cultural in their representations of nontraditional kinship and identity by focusing on the moments where the formulaic genre logic may be troubled by a representation of lived experience that exceeds the scope of the heterocoital framework tropes. For example, the value of heterocoital family is consistently reaffirmed through heterocoital family plots, which have also become the telos of most mass-market nontraditional kinship films. However, family configurations engendered by non-heterocoital reproduction and kinship may exceed the range of culturally available affective scripts for processing matters of kinship that are typically encoded in the heterocoital nuclear family plot. Another variable is the positionality of specific viewers. Adoption, in particular, is one of the social relationships that lead to experiences that cannot be construed definitively as either beneficial or harmful, either to the individuals involved or to the social order. And so, depending on positionality, the viewers' reactions to representations of adoption and nontraditional kinship in film may vary. While viewers who take heterocoital reproduction and identity for granted may feel reassured by a reaffirmation of heterocoital family and origin, lived experiences of nontraditional reproduction participants may cause a range of reactions to such reaffirmations. The peripeteia of nontraditional reproduction plots that still serve to highlight the primacy of heterocoital family as a linchpin of human nature can be experienced as othering by someone whose origin and kinship are thus construed as reproductive difference. The logic of heterocoital reproduction narrative representation may misrepresent nontraditional reproduction experiences and make them unrecognizable and objectionable to those who know the subject intimately.

Analysis in this book takes into account the range of viewer's responses to representation of nontraditional reproduction and kinship, but the main object of analysis is most often what Müller and Kappelhoff call the "spectator-I," which is different from the "empirical viewer" (51). They describe the spectator-I as "a specific positioning of the viewer," an "implicit or ideal spectator" who would experience the film via "complete saturation in the semiotic material or even authorial intention" (51). In other words, from such a position, all the intended effects of the film would be experienced by the viewer exactly as they were intended by film creators. This position may be but does not have to be occupied by every empirical, actual viewer. For example, an adoptee or a birth parent may experience emotions incongruent with those intended in a portrayal of adoption as salvation. Since the spectator-I is "a theoretical position of agency that might be taken by an empirical subject" (92), it is through this position that fictional narratives may be connected to the social. Either by inhabiting the position of the spectator-I or by experiencing oneself as its "other," the viewer participates in the creation of shared reality. The production of shared reality, according to Müller and Kappelhoff, happens when a "narrative emerges from the viewer's experiential engagement with movement-images in a process of 'fictionalization'" (27), which can be understood as "'as-if-I-were-interacting-with-a-reality-surrounding-me'" (38). The "as-if" quality means that "*for the moment of their reception,* [spectators] *replace* [their everyday reality] *by an apparent reality*" (38). It is at this moment that the culturally sanctioned narrative may be affectively anchored in the viewer's mind and become the basis for value judgments. In the context of adoption and ARTs, cinematic narratives become reference points for individual personal connections to affective scripts for experiencing and processing nontraditional reproduction and kinship information. In this way, the film aesthetic may facilitate affective acculturation to the normativity in nontraditional reproduction.

Typically, the primacy of heterocoital reproduction, identity, and kinship is reconfirmed in film as formative of the shared reality. But the "objectivity" of such reality, according to Sara Ahmed, "is an effect rather than a cause" of affect circulation (10). Sara Ahmed's theory of "sociality of emotions" (10) argues that emotions are not private properties or states of an individual but rather the means by which an individual and the collective "are delineated as if they were objects" (10). Such objectification constitutes a relationship of belonging between an individual and the collective. According to Ahmed, "emotions provide a script" that makes the formation of "I" possible through feeling a certain way about certain others, which becomes a condition of belonging (12). In other words, if you feel *x* (about *z*), you are one of *y*. This process relies on fetishization of emotions, through which the "history of their production and circulation" (11) is erased in order to establish "the psychic and social as objects" (10) "saturated with affect" (11) that can then be circulated to facilitate "invest[ment] in social norms" (12). Such affective attachments to social norms and categories fix the subjects within structures that perpetuate "conditions of . . . subordination," and emotion becomes "a form of cultural politics or world making" (12). The social structures, in turn, "become sticky, or saturated with affect, as sites of personal and social tension" to the point that "their demise is felt as a kind of living death" (Ahmed 11, 12). Heterocoital family and origin, for instance, are such structures in the context of adoption and ARTs.

It is important to recognize that if we follow Ahmed and Müller and Kappelhoff, we are moving away from understanding texts as mere scripts for affect or culturally sanctioned behavior and toward seeing them as a means of producing in the viewer or reader a historically specific affective experience, which results in a historically and culturally specific shared reality that determines the kinds of subjects, objects of feeling, and relationships of belonging that are possible at this historical moment. In other words, texts are conduits of "structures of feeling"—a term Raymond Williams coined in order to "correlate material, social, and affective structures" (Sharma and Tygstrup 2). In *Preface to Film,* Williams and Orrom consider structures of feeling as the ineffable element of the "living experience of the time" (21) encoded in the artistic "conventions—the means of expression which find tacit consent" or "accepted standard" (22, 23). For example, realism in film may mean not only "verisimilitude in representation" but also a correspondence to the contemporaneous "ideas of 'normality' and of 'probability'" (30). Within this framework, *realistic* means "being part of normal everyday experience of those by and for whom the film is made" as well as being "psychologically convincing and true" (29, 30). Like novels, films may also be "believable stories that [do] not solicit belief" (Gallagher 340). The "reality" of cinematic representation depends on the ability of the audience to recognize the logic of the art form. Among other things, such recognition is facilitated by genre.

Cultural values, generic conventions, and human emotional affordances come together to produce "orientations," in Ahmed's sense, of the viewers "towards the objects that are identified as their cause" (Ahmed 13). Genre conventions, specifically, encode the structures of feeling appropriate to specific contexts, and they can be understood, albeit in a limited way, through analysis of representational logic and cinematic techniques. By looking at the ways nontraditional reproduction is conceptualized and represented in different film genres, it is possible to see what structures of feeling support cultural ideas about identity, kinship, and belonging and how our attachment to these ideas is fostered through film-viewing experiences. With an implicit understanding that affective orientations are not just a private matter, film criticism has treated genre analysis as a social practice. According to Rick Altman, "genres are never neutral categories" and "they—and their critics and theorists—always participate in and further the work of various institutions" by anchoring both pleasure from the socially acceptable and contempt for the marginalized (12). Susan Merrill Squier evokes Tony Bennett's genre theory that considers genres "as nodes of social practices" and "part[s] of the set of networked relations—relations that extend all across the social field from the material to the semiotic" (21). Anis Bawarshi claims that "typified texts reflect and reproduce social situations and activities" (336) and, as Squier explains, serve as "both . . . regulatory and . . . constitutive category[ies]," as they "shap[e] how a preexisting social practice can be entered and engaged in" while at the same time they build up this practice by "giving us the conventions that make it possible for us to enact that practice" (Bawarshi, ctd. in Squier 21). The common ground between these scholars is that genres are both reflective and formative of social practices, and therefore they can serve as sources of established cultural ideas that underpin our social lives.

The difficulty of categorizing films into genres is commonly stated in film studies. While some genres, such as the western and film noir, have been established and widely studied, it is also often apparent that a film can be a genre hybrid or genres can be understood as modes. Comedic or melodramatic elements, for example, may be present across genres. And yet, marketing genre designations target the viewers' expectations of specific modes of viewing experience, and labeling a film as an instance of a genre lets prospective consumers know what "story and the kind of pleasure it [is] likely to offer" (Grant 2012, xviii). While some scholars, like Altman, consider genres historically specific, others, like Torben Grodal, believe that genres harness universal "cognitive and emotional competencies" (45) of a regular viewer. For Altman, such response is "Pavlovian": it relies on the viewer's familiarity with conventions and is achieved by the viewer's gradual immersion in the film by accepting the "genre cue[s]" (151). Grodal attributes generic pleasure to a film's tapping into primordial basic emotions, "such as fear, love, lust, or sadness" (54). According to Grodal, a viewer may have a genre-expected reaction to the film without knowing its genre due to the universality of certain emotion and situation "bundles" (55). He observes that such bundles may elicit similar reactions in the viewers of different cultures; for example, one of the bundles—"attachment between children and parents"—"ha[s] a universal core that supports the spread of mind-grabbing cultural products" (55). Genres thus become "prototype[s]" (Grodal, 44) recognizable across contexts.[15] In either case, the generic pleasure is evoked in the viewer by activating intended emotional responses to events, dialogues, and characters, and these theories are not necessarily mutually exclusive. For example, horror films rely on archetypal fear-inducing narratives and situations, which may be specified as a script that reflects contemporaneous historical conditions and culture-specific values.

While it may seem that adoption and ARTs cinema informs the culture about nontraditional reproduction or is reflecting cultural ideas about it, this book argues that popular genre cinema is primarily concerned with shoring up the cultural primacy of the heterocoital family, even as it is portraying adoption and ARTs. Cultural ideas about nontraditional reproduction still tend to be ideas about "the other" of the heterocoital family that serve to boost its cultural importance by emphasizing the as-ifness of non-heterocoital reproduction. The films discussed in this book are not aimed specifically at the audience that may have a more direct, and therefore nuanced, involvement with nontraditional reproduction. Unlike documentaries authored by adoptees or independent films, these popular culture cinematic texts may forgo a nuanced representation of nontraditional kinship practices in favor of engaging with the more culturally palatable representations that can range from the blatantly threatening "other," to the "other" domesticated through the metaphor of the heterocoital family. The former explicitly insists on heterocoital normativity. But in the latter's case, the viewer that lacks personal experience with nontraditional reproduction may develop a stance of acceptance toward the domesticated other by imagining them through the cultural scripts that regulate the heterocoital family and in this way still participate in unintended epistemological erasure of alternative ways of being. In either process, the viewer is acculturated to the idea that nontraditional reproduction has to

15. Robert Warshow's definition of genre as "a system of conventions structured according to cultural values" is yet another way to understand the terms of the viewer's relationship with film (Grant 2012, xviii).

conform to the heterocoital script, and in this way the oppressive character of reproductive difference may be solidified.[16]

The interconnected social, affective, and aesthetic structures are stable enough to hold the fabric of reality together, but not rigid. In order to account for challenges to heterocoital reproductive order that may result in cultural changes, this book points to the moments of genres' failures to pull us into the intended affective script. These moments make visible the contours of both the normative and the alternative possibilities for the lived experience of reproduction. In the space of contact between the movement-image focused by a spectator-I and the empirical viewer's experience of viewing the film (informed by their own lived experience), the change of formal art conventions and structures of feeling anticipated by Williams may happen, and "meaning-making in cinematic metaphor [may] thus becom[e] the joint sharing of an *always changing* reality" (Müller and Kappelhoff 79; emphasis mine). In such moments, we can notice that adoption and ARTs trouble established ways of life, even if they imitate heterocoital scripts or heterosexual ways of kinship. Depending on our epistemological stance, we might see nontraditional families as "passing" for heterocoital ones, or we may notice that we expect reproduction of heterosexual culture in visibly nontraditional families. The viewers' experience of such negotiation between heterocoital and nontraditional reproduction may gradually veer toward hybridization of cultural scripts for kinship, even if a film ends in a reaffirmation of the heterocoital order. Such experience is not a simple substitution or subjection of the new script to the old. Rather, if we view a film critically and we know what to look for, heterocoital reproduction becomes visible as a metaphor for thinking about new kinds of reproduction and kinship. In other words, the viewer

16. If the affective response suggested by a film feels inorganic, the result is experiences of exclusion, inadequacy, not being seen and understood, a lack of voice. But instead of disruptions, these experiences may still serve to further reinforce heterocoital frameworks. For example, people who have had a lived experience of adoption might experience such discomfort when watching films about adoption. Gailey is writing about a strong reaction to Spielberg's *A.I.* by adoptees, many of whom did not think the film was successful in portraying "what [adoptees] are really like" (84). Susan Bordo observes that adoption cinema tends to represent birth parents in ways that all parties to adoption may experience as troubling. Such discomfort is rarely the experience of those viewers who only have had experiences of normative reproduction and kinship, which suggests that mass-market adoption and ARTs film may not normalize adoptive and nontraditional reproduction community, even though it seems to broaden public awareness of the phenomenon and acculturate the normative society to the non-heterocoital ways of life. This is not to say that everyone who is "normative" would have a seamless experience watching an adoption film, but the sense of ease is more likely to be approximated by such viewers, since most nontraditional reproduction films are aimed at mass-market audiences that uphold heterocoital reproductive norms as an ideal to which all lived experience ought to conform.

may become aware that they are challenged to experience one thing in terms of another (e.g., an adoptive family in terms of heterocoital family), and in the process of such hybridization, the position of the heterocoital reproduction script as the *only* one may be incrementally eroded.

•

The chapters of this book examine reaffirmations and challenges to the heterocoital order through specific affective landscapes of drama, comedy, horror, and sci-fi. The scope is limited to these four genres due to their popularity and in the interest of space, so children's cinema and superhero films, for example, are not considered in this book, even though adoption is featured prominently in them. While sci-fi is not the most popular genre, the book begins and ends with discussions of sci-fi films because this genre is dealing explicitly with representations of technologies and their impact on visions of the future. Due to its attention to human-technology enmeshments, it paves the way toward the discussion of critical posthumanist thought in the conclusion as a methodology for thinking about reproduction in further research. As a speculative genre, sci-fi offers a unique kind of representation, since it imagines possible scenarios of integrating new reproductive technologies and adoption through the current cultural ideas about the subject, thus exposing potential alignments with and challenges to the heterocoital symbolic order. At the same time, the fictional aspect of sci-fi allows for a safe exploration of nontraditional reproduction's potential to reinvent culture. This genre makes visible cultural anxieties and expectations attached to the new reproductive possibilities, but "the denial of truth inherent in fiction" helps us "protect ourselves from acknowledging [our repressed impulses and desires], and from having to deal with their consequences" (Squier 18). Recently, sci-fi, which used to be a genre concerned with future projections, has been increasingly perceived as a genre that coproduces reality. Squier observes "a shift in the social valuation of science fiction" that reverses the ethos of the genre commonly understood as science-represented-in-fiction (19). The reversal enables fiction to change technosocial reality; for example, "the transformative processes of biomedicine are enabled somehow by the transformative narrative that is science fiction" (19). Sherryl Vint, too, claims that sci-fi narrative analysis is a practice of understanding not only how it represents science and technology but also what it aims to manifest, speculate into being. According to Vint, "science fiction has moved from being a niche genre at the beginning of the twentieth century to a widely shared cultural vernacular for describing the twenty-first" (55). She claims that sci-fi narratives produce "affective attachments" to "visions of possible futures" as a way to "marshal attention and energy to projects, nurturing them into materiality or resisting their arrival" (53). In other words, sci-fi has become the grounds for understanding technology as shaping shared reality, and affective responses to futuristic scenarios have transcended the fictional realm and have acquired world-building power. On the one hand, sci-fi domesticates the unknown by thinking through possibilities that tantalize popular imagination in response to scientific discoveries. On the other hand, sci-fi is the genre that challenges heterocoital scripts further than the more conservative genres of drama, horror, and comedy discussed in chapters 1, 2, and 3. The visibility of the challenge makes cultural resistance and co-optation of the new possibilities also more visible and available for analysis.

Chapter 1 concerns itself with nontraditional reproduction drama, which registers narratives that are accepted as "real," that is, narratives that explore believable human stories. It tends to focus on an individual's journey and mostly relies on tropes of rescue (adoption), search and reunion (adoption and ARTs), and pursuit of fertility (ARTs). Drama relies on emotions associated with sympathy and relief in response to sadness triggered by the topics of family separation, loss, redemption, and salvation. This chapter establishes one of the main ideas of this book—adoption and ART narratives reinscribe heterocoital imaginaries even as they present nontraditional forms of kinship and reproduction.

Horror (chapter 2) and comedy (chapter 3) are interested in the influence of adoption and ARTs on the community and explore a person's origin as a force that challenges communal ways. Both genres are conservative, although comedy is less so, and, like drama, are concerned with reestablishing the heterocoital origin script or a more successful imitation of it. Both comedy and horror stage mayhem that upends the existing social order only to restore it in the happy ending. Horror builds up fear and disgust and resolves the plot conflict in a pleasurable vanquishing of the monster, thus rejecting unacceptable ways of being. The pleasure attached to comedic peripeteia leaves more room for imagining alternative ways and forms of life and belonging. For example, the excess of queer characters and situations, and potential viewers' pleasurable responses to them, destabilizes heterosexuality as a natural condition and a means of reproduction, which exposes and questions a link between biogenetic reproduction and heterosexual culture transfer. In this way, adoption and ART comedy disturbs heterocoital order even as it reliably leads the viewer to a heterosexual union in the happy ending, coupled with a reaffirmation if the heterocoital family. Both chapters introduce further reflections on the significance of challenges presented by ARTs to the heterocoital order and show that these challenges are a threat to the whole paradigm of heteropatriarchy. Analysis of ART films in these chapters shows that reproductive technologies open space for a renegotiation of men's and women's reproductive power. Plot outcomes in the films discussed trend toward assuaging patriarchy's anxieties through reestablishing control over the woman's reproductive capacity or doing away with the need for a female in the process altogether.

The conclusion of the book expands on the idea that anxieties over challenges to the heterocoital order are anxieties over the stability of the patriarchy's control over reproduction and kinship making. Since at the core of the heterocoital and heterosexual order is the patriarchal control over the woman's body, its reproductive function, and children, technological changes to the reproductive process may bring into play new forms of power. The conclusion reflects on such possibilities and shows that possible outcomes of technological development may emerge as patriarchal futures that erase the reproductive power of the woman by making the reproductive female body unnecessary or dehumanized as a reproductive machine, or, alternatively, as the breakdown of patriarchal control over reproduction, which may mean a new kind of freedom, a new conceptualization of the relationship between humans and technology, and a new stance toward the world. Reproductive technology development demands a cultural response, and the conclusion of this book invites further reflection on reproductive futurities through nondualistic and post-anthropocentric thinking paradigms. To that end, the conclusion discusses the importance of posthumanist thought in reconceptualizing reproduction imaginaries.

While the main thrust of this book's argument is a critique of the heterocoital imaginary and ideology as a foundation of patriarchy, the book is not advocating the erasure of the nuclear heterocoital family. We need to keep in mind that access to heterocoital family and biogenetic reproduction is a site of inequality and struggle for reproductive justice. Access to heterocoital family has been weaponized against specific groups through slavery, Native American genocide, the Page Act of 1975, disability and same-sex discourses, et cetera. For many, this way of family making is an expression of freedom, inclusion, and biocultural continuity. Yet another concern may emerge if we stop normalizing nontraditional reproductive origin through heterocoital scripts without a radical revision of anthropocentric dualisms: reproductive difference as a distinction between who is produced by heterocoitus and who is a product of technogenesis may become institutionalized as a vector of oppression. If left unexamined, the difference in (biogenetic) origin may lead to the creation of a social category of reproductive difference—between "naturally" and "artificially" reproduced humans. The contours of the human, which have never been clear and always exclusionary, may be blurred further along the line of the (so far) most stable definition as a reproductive biological species. The definition of "[the] human" in the *Oxford English Dictionary* is telling in that it aims to delineate the human as not divine, machine, or animal. Most of the definitions under the noun and adjective entries are tautological (human is what humans do), and only one definition remains more or less straightforward and grounded—that of the biological species, *Homo sapiens*. New reproductive technologies threaten to blur the boundaries even of this definition and make the term even more contingent on broad social consensus about what it means to be human. One of the ways to deal with this new problem may be following the familiar path: developing an awareness of the new form of difference and then focusing on inclusion of reproductive diversity under the umbrella of the new expanded definition of humanity. But such inclusion will still be happening on the terms of the dualistic, anthropocentric, and likely patriarchal paradigm, by exclusion of yet another "other." Alternatively, a "reproductive consciousness" (to borrow a term from Mary O'Brien [1981, 27]) informed by critical posthumanism—a mode of postdualistic thinking—could accept technogenesis as a constitutive feature of humanity. Such reframing would call for a reexamination of the worldview built on dualisms-informed hierarchies in order to think beyond the divide between humans and technology and its role in distinguishing between "real" and "not real" humans and kinships. Revisions of binary and anthropocentric views of the world suggested by critical posthumanism can help conceive of future social and cultural structures that support all forms of identities, belonging, and ways of life that can affirm everyone's existence regardless of their reproductive identity. Such vision demands a new cultural imaginary for living with difference without oppression. Rethinking reproduction may offer a way in.

CHAPTER 1

Adoption and ARTs in (Melo)Drama

The Two Mothers Problem

> The ideology of monomaternalism, like the ideology of monogamy, promotes practices that uphold the heteropatriarchal nuclear family.
>
> —Shelley M. Park, *Mothering Queerly, Queering Motherhood* (6)

> SADIE (gamete donor): Do you think our baby will grow up to be a writer?
>
> RACHEL (gamete recipient): Yours and Sam's?
>
> SADIE: No, yours and mine.
>
> —*Private Life*

The genre of melodrama itself is typically driven by tensions between what is socially acceptable and what is not, and the affective arc of such narrative is moving the viewer from the sense of being morally injured toward satisfaction with justice served. The pleasure viewers take in the happy ending is tied to socially desirable outcomes. While melodrama is notoriously amorphous as a genre and is often considered as a mode that may be present in other genres, the common specific quality of melodramatic affective landscape is the tension created by the struggle between good and evil. Melodramatic imagination, according to Peter Brooks, is producing "the drama of morality" that aims to reaffirm "the existence of a moral universe" against the obstacles mounted by "villainy and perversions of judgment" (20). Dramas are not unequivocally didactic, though. E. Deidre Pribram accounts for conflicts that expose tensions between social mores and characters' desires by claiming that "a melodramatic vision [is] focused on culturally embedded beings operating within or contesting social institutions and practices" (2018, 237). She sees the cultural value of melodrama in its excess of emotionality, which, if accepted as an aesthetic feature, can reveal "processes, meanings, and *social purposes* of emotional life" (237; emphasis mine). Christine Gledhill also sees melodrama as a "repositor[y] of emotional knowledge," and the purpose of melodrama's "oppositional protagonists" in manifesting both "emerging feelings and perceptions" and the "residual and dominant structures of feeling" against which the new ways of thinking and feeling become visible (2018, xxiv). Beyond the emotions exchanged by characters on the screen, the affective experiences of the viewers can tell us about which new ways of being and feeling are butting against which culturally acceptable affective scripts. In the case of cinema portraying adoption and other nontraditional kinship, melodramatic genre reveals cultural negotiations around the connections between forms of reproduction and kinship, origin, identity, and belonging.

The second epigraph to this chapter comes from Tamara Jenkins's film *Private Life,* which tells a story of an infertile heterosexual couple trying to start a family either through adoption or ARTs. This tidbit of dialogue happens while Rachel's niece is undergoing a fertility treatment to produce viable eggs for her aunt to use in a cycle of IVF. Sadie's last remark is met with a bewildered silence on the part of Rachel, who realizes the complications such arrangement might bring into her and her husband Paul's life. A quote from a flyer about egg donation given to Rachel by her fertility doctor—"Sometimes it takes three to make a family"—acquires a new meaning. Up to this point, Rachel has been thinking of egg donation as if it were a closed adoption: by bracketing out the relatives exceeding the heterosexual reproduction dyad, it creates an appearance of a heterocoital nuclear family. Non-anonymous egg donation, though, seems to be closer to an open adoption. Sadie imagines the process as collaboration. She speaks as if she will have some degree of child ownership in this arrangement and the child will have two mothers. The lack of expanded kinship vocabulary to accommodate a social arrangement that involves three parties in biogenetic reproduction gives Rachel pause. This scene from *Private Life* is representative of plot conflicts in adoption and ARTs melodrama.[1]

Overall, nontraditional reproduction melodramas contribute to the persistence of heterocoital frameworks by imagining all family formations through the metaphor of the heterocoital nuclear family. In fact, adoption and ART melodramas are not primarily concerned with nontraditional reproduction matters, even if they may be the focal point of the plot. Rather, like many other genres, melodrama uses adoption and other forms of nontraditional

1. Melodrama is understood here not as musical drama (the term's original meaning) but, in Peter Brooks's terms, "a mode of high emotionalism and stark ethical conflict" (12). Peter Brooks distinguishes between melodrama, a mode "intermediate between tragedy and comedy—but explicitly not a mixture of the two" and "naturalistic 'realism'" (13). The melodramatic mode, according to him, aims not to represent reality "truthfully" but to "exploit the dramatics and excitement discoverable within the real, to heighten in dramatic gesture the moral crises and peripeties of life" (13). The terms *melodrama* and *drama* will be used interchangeably.

reproduction as plot devices to explore and neutralize threats they present to the heterocoital order. Commercially successful nontraditional reproduction melodrama is invested in reaffirming heterocoital kinship norms by educating the viewer in ways of feeling the right way about different kinds of families. By exalting the heterocoital family, nontraditional reproduction melodrama helps maintain the order within which "patriarchy, compulsory heterosexuality, white supremacy, and socioeconomic inequality are actively *reproduced* through the social and legal construction of legitimate families" (Patton-Imani 13). Adoption narratives may reinforce the heterocoital framework even when they represent adoption as a socially sanctioned reproductive choice. To maintain the primacy of the heterocoital family, nontraditional reproduction may be represented as a form of suffering or a "second-best" option that prospective parents agonize over even though they are "doing the right thing." Alternatively, it may be celebrated as a good *imitation* of heterocoital family. This chapter will show that even though cultural standards for legitimacy of families may be challenged by representations of nontraditional reproduction, the cultural commitment to heterocoital family persists and "few dare to reject the biological model that sustains the judicially created family" (Modell 5).

Adoption as a theme lends itself especially well to the Manichean logic of melodramatic imagination. Its archetypal narrative types include, for example, "adoption as rescue," which centers on the adoptive family. In this scenario, adoptive parents rescue an endangered child, and, more recently, the child might also rescue the parents emotionally. Another type of narrative is the search and reunion plot, which centers on adoptees and biological parents looking for each other. In search and reunion adoption narratives, biogenetic bonds may heal not only searching adoptees or their biogenetic parents but also adoptive families. After the adoptee's need for origin knowledge is satisfied, they can reinstate their kinship connections with the adoptive family. And, finally, there is the ripped-from-the-headlines scenario of birth parents claiming the adopted child back. This one often engages with the same insecurities about child ownership in the adoptive family that are negotiated in the search and rescue scenario, but here such insecurities are not the corollary of the adoptee's search but the central conflict. The focus is less on the adoptee's desires, since the adoptee is typically a young child, and more on a competition between the adoptive and biological parents' rights to the child. In addition to adoption plots, a common ART plot might involve fertility struggles of a couple, which may or may not end in reproductive success. In such narratives, adoption may be involved as a secondary plotline. All narrative types negotiate the cultural hierarchy of heterocoital and nontraditional families through the logic of duality in which one of the elements is preferable. For instance, even though the outcomes of such narratives may be a reaffirmation of the validity of the adoptive family, the presence of the birth family and the emotional struggle involved in "overcoming" the power of the searching adoptee's bond with their birth parents serves as a reminder of its cultural primacy. The above scenarios are often engaged by melodrama in a dualistic way, pitting the nontraditional and heterocoital kin against each other in the struggle over the ownership of the child or the adult adopted person's choice of affiliation.

Two of the films considered in this chapter—*Losing Isaiah* (1995) and *Mother and Child* (2010)—provide interesting case studies in adoption melodrama and the ways it negotiates kinship configurations that exceed the heterocoital framework. Both films explore nontraditional family making against the kinship logic of the heterocoital family (in addition to adoption, there is single motherhood and interracial kinship), and both negotiate culturally acceptable reproduction and kinship through the process of figuring out whom the adopted children belong *to* and belong *with*. Race in these films serves as a visible marker of the biological, heterocoital origin, which ultimately determines socially acceptable kinship. *Losing Isaiah* follows the "birth mother as a threat" scenario, familiar to the viewers as an archetypal media story. *Mother and Child* weaves a more complex narrative of genealogical and affective entanglements. Yet, in the end, both films affirm the primacy of the heterocoital family and the cultural idea that unconditional parental love is linked to the "natural"—in other words, biogenetic—bond.

Losing Isaiah follows a dispute between a Black biological mother and a white family who adopted her child. It follows the "logic of the excluded middle," that is, the polarization of stances, outcomes, and characters, presented as a conflict between good and evil (Brooks 18). The film is set in Chicago during the crack epidemic of the early 1980s through the early 1990s. Khaila (Halle Berry) stashes her newborn baby, Isaiah, in a box in an alley and goes looking for drugs. When she comes back, the child is gone. He was discovered by a trash pickup crew just before they were about to throw the box into the trash compactor. Isaiah ends up in a hospital, where Margaret Lewin (Jessica Lange), a social worker, takes care of him and ultimately decides to foster and adopt the boy. Margaret lives with her husband, Charlie (David Strathairn), and her daughter, Hannah (Daisy Eagan)—a typical suburban white middle-class family. Isaiah (Marc John Jefferies) stays with the Lewins for three years. During this time, Khaila is recovering from drug abuse and, with the help of her caseworker, discovers that Isaiah is alive. They hire a lawyer (Samuel L. Jackson) to contest the adoption. The court returns Isaiah to Khaila, but she has trouble dealing with his emotional outbursts, caused by his separation

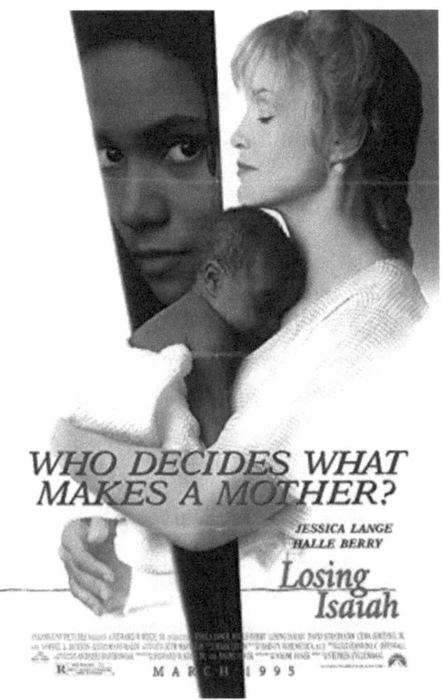

FIGURE 1.1. *Losing Isaiah* poster. Paramount Pictures, 1995.

from the adoptive family. She invites Margaret to be a part of Isaiah's transition, and in the final scene, both women play building blocks with Isaiah at his school.

The binary nature of the film's conflict is represented quite obviously in the design of the film's release poster (see figure 1.1), which shows Lange-Margaret with a Black baby, staged as Madonna and child. She is an angelic blonde, placed against white background. The baby's head is cradled comfortably in the curve of her neck. She is looking down with her eyes peacefully closed as if her gaze is directed inward, and she is fully focused on the child. Berry-Khaila is looking at them from a dark rip in the white fabric of the background; she is looking sideways, intensely. Her image is meant to evoke a feeling of impending danger that lurks in the shadows. The poster suggests a competitive dichotomy between the birth and adoptive mothers and points to the idea of the biological mother as a threat to the adoptive mother and child bond. The baby is in the center of the image. His placement in the arms of Margaret may suggest his belonging with the saint-like figure in the foreground. He is wrapped in a white blanket that connects him to the white background and suggests care provided by the adoptive mother. But the color of his skin blends in with the dark background that hides Khaila's body, and the dark rip in the white space invokes the power of his biological origin to trouble the connection that is built through nurture. Margaret's forearm, which hugs the baby and connects the edges of the dark gash in the white background, seems to be the only thing that holds the ripped space apart. The inscription on the release poster asks, "Who decides what makes a mother?" underscoring the dichotomy at the center of the film's conflict.

Losing Isaiah belongs to the "wave" of films "about adoption, foster care, and the relative 'fitness' or otherwise of poor and middle-class mothers" that, according to Sandra Patton, "began appearing in the spring of 1994" in response to public discussion and legislation on transracial adoption in 1993 and 1994 (132). The negotiation of the child's belonging that is central to the plot of the film represents the tension between the African American community's resistance to interracial adoptions, expressed in the 1972 position statement by the National Association of Black Social Workers (NABSW), and the push to curtail the racial and ethnic matching policies that led to the passing of the Multiethnic Placement Act (MEPA) in 1994, Interethnic Placement Act (IEPA) in 1996, and Adoption and Safe Families Act (ASFA) in 1997. These legislative acts aimed to remove barriers to interracial, international, and intercultural adoption; adoption agencies that would not follow nonmatching policies risked the loss of federal funds. NABSW's objection to interracial placements cited concerns over the ability of white adoptive parents to provide transracial adoptees organic access to African American culture and to equip transracial adoptees with the social skills necessary for navigating a racist society. The 1972 position statement was reinforced by the NABSW in 1991 and in their 1994 *Preserving African American Families,* which was a call to curb interracial adoptions (ctd. in Griffith and Bergeron 305). NABSW's statements protested the removal of African American children from homes deemed unsafe and the resulting demonization of Black families, which intensified during the crack epidemic, as represented in *Losing Isaiah.*[2] The "crack baby epidemic" narrative was eventually discredited after several studies had failed to find a connection between mothers' crack use and possible birth defects or cognitive deficits in babies. More generally, the resistance to separating Black children from their biological parents has been fueled by the slavery-inflected history of exploiting Black bodies as a resource for white domesticity.[3]

The film has been consistently understood as a response to this contemporaneous social climate. Sandra Patton, for example, reads *Losing Isaiah* as a type of story characteristic of the crack baby epidemic era and its aftermath.

2. For a more detailed discussion of the crack epidemic and its connection to legislation and policies regulating reproduction and kinship, see Patton; Ortiz and Briggs (esp. 44–46).

3. For a detailed discussion of this history see Roberts (2022).

She notices "the congruence of the messages in *Losing Isaiah* with the conservative politics of the moment" (135) that imagine Black families as "destroyed by the 'culture of poverty'" from which "innocent children must be saved" by "white nuclear families, possessors of 'family values'" (133). Such stories solicit public support for legislative decisions that legitimize removal of children from Black parents deemed unfit and their adoption by white families. Patton explains that in order to build a moral justification for such legislation, "Black children are [represented as] uncared-for and unwanted by their Black families, and thus must be saved by those fit to save, and redeem these lost children—White women" (133). Susan Bordo also observes that the white savior trope frames the film's plot, which presents Margaret, the white adoptive mother, as a "saver of babies that others have discarded, the solid, whole, mirror image of the cracked one: Isaiah's birth mom" (327). This seems to be, indeed, the stance of the Lewins, who feel entitled to keep Isaiah because his mother is "a junkie" who put her son in the garbage. In a direct confrontation with Khaila in the court bathroom, Margaret says, "Any animal can give birth. That doesn't make it a mother," implying that Khaila's lack of nurturing ability makes her unfit to mother. Moments like this may lead to reading *Losing Isaiah* as one of the films that portray the adoptive mother as more "competent" than the birth mother (Bordo 326) and thus endorse the white adoptive mother's "colorblind concept of raising children, which the film clearly applauds" (327).

Losing Isaiah does have enough scenes that promote color-blind reasoning and the idea that the right kind of affect and nurture is what makes a family real. The most often-cited scene shows Lewin's biological daughter, Hannah, playing with Isaiah. They are comfortably positioned in the bathroom, a space suggesting intimacy, and it is also the right place to blow bubbles. Isaiah is excited as he is trying to catch them; he is clearly happy. In the middle of the game, Hannah catches one of his hands and asks, "Look at our hands—what's different about them?" Isaiah replies, "My hand is smaller," avoiding the obvious comment about different skin color. Margaret reinforces this argument in her court testimony when she counters the question about Isaiah's lack of access to African American history and culture by asking, "What about love?" She demonstrates a lack of awareness of the racial context even more egregiously when she says to Khaila during their confrontation in the bathroom, "All you people think about is color." Besides its obvious racism, Margaret's comment is a rejection of the importance of race and biological origin to Isaiah's best interests and an argument for the right to parent based on affect and nurture, not the biological connection. But Margaret's argument is not quite the film's argument. When exasperated Margaret says to the lawyer, "But I am his mother!" the lawyer quips, "Are you?" Khaila counters Margaret's color blindness by calling out her use of "you people" and reminding her that she and Isaiah are "the same kind of people." The white adoption agency worker questioned in court testifies that their policy is to match adoptees and adoptive families, and the recommendation is to return the child to the biological mother. She responds to the objection that it takes a long time to find a Black adoptive family (a typical argument for MEPA) by protesting the idea that taking a child away from poor Black parents for a placement with a well-off white family is in the child's best interest. "What kind of values does that suggest?" she asks and reminds the audience that the long-term best interest of the child in this case would be to stay with his biological mother, who can provide both a model for racial identification and adequate care.

The film presents Khaila as becoming such a mother. While the beginning of the film does portray her briefly as a stereotypical crack user, unconcerned with the well-being of her child, over the course of the film, the viewer witnesses her transformation into a loving and capable mother. She is shown as a recovering drug addict, a responsible caregiver, and a decent woman who refuses advances of a married man. Her transformation starts with a confession. While reading a book about a woman who got pregnant, Khaila admits to her social worker that she "threw [her son] away." She breaks down as she starts reading a passage about the woman's visit to the doctor, who tells her not to drink alcohol or take medicine and eat healthy so her baby could "grow strong." We witness Khaila's regret and shame as she tells the social worker that she killed her baby. This repentance seems to be provoked by a passage about good mothering, which names for the viewer the change in her: she understands now what it is to be a good mother and that she has not been a good one. Her competence as a caregiver is demonstrated in working as a nanny for a white family and in taking care of the children of the woman from whom she rents a room. When her landlady, Marie, is annoyed by her son Amir, Khaila tells her it's wrong. When Marie is taken to the hospital with a miscarriage, she stays with Marie's children and takes care of them. She resists the temptation to smoke the crack she finds in Marie's bed and remains a stabilizing presence for Amir and his sister. While some of Khaila's transformation is prompted by her lawyer, who aims to present her as a credible parent, the film shows Khaila becoming one even before she gets an apartment of her own, wears feminine outfits and pearls, and starts going to church. Her virtue is further confirmed when she refuses advances from Eddie (Cuba Gooding Jr.) until he initiates a divorce from his former wife. The result of Khaila's transformation is her credibility as a mother in the eyes of the court, where she shows her remorse and testifies to a higher power helping her turn around and stay good.

Taken as a whole, the film hardly seems to endorse unequivocally the white savior trope, the competency of the white mother, or a color-blind attitude. Rather, it lends itself to polarizing readings that may favor one side of the typical arguments in the debate about interracial adoption that are constitutive of the plot's central conflict. Even when the film tries to introduce nuance in the binary thinking about who deserves to be Isaiah's mother, the two sides of the argument mostly clash without changing each other, which prompts the viewer to take a side in a complex situation where taking a side seems impossible. The conversations Khaila and the Lewins have with their lawyers show the complexities of their positionality against the kinship ideology that encourages binary choices. Kadar Lewis (Samuel L. Jackson), a lawyer whom Khaila hires in order to contest adoption on the grounds she was not informed about it, takes on pro bono "socially relevant" cases that can "set legal precedent." The lawyer is not convinced of Khaila's ability to leave the drugs behind, but he thinks that her case "fits [the] profile" he is looking for. While he is skeptical that she can be a good mother to Isaiah, he believes that winning her case would help the cause of keeping Black families together. For him, Khaila's case has significance beyond this specific adoption or even beyond getting justice for Black mothers affected by the supposed crack baby crisis. His agenda aligns with the 1991 statement by NABSW, and to him, "this goes way beyond [Khaila]. Black babies belong with Black mothers." In Lewis's opinion, the case is tough because the adoptive "family is white," and they have been providing good care for Isaiah. When Khaila is trying to object—"But I'm his mother!"—Lewis replies that he is sure that the adoptive mother thinks this as well, as do many other people. In response to Khaila's reliance on the biological tie, he points out the importance of parental competence and appropriate affect, which the court and popular opinion will take into account when deciding who deserves to be a parent. Lewis draws attention to the social aspect of kinship, which may trump Khaila's biological connection given the lapse in her adherence to socially acceptable motherhood.

Yet, just when the film seems to suggest the importance of nurture in the parenthood debate, it reintroduces arguments based on the significance of the biological bond. Charlie and Margaret also talk to a lawyer—Caroline Jones (LaTanya Richardson). Jones is a Black attorney who counters their indignation at the "junkie" who has no right to the abandoned child with a firm statement that Khaila has the right to be heard. The lawyer warns the Lewins that the court may reverse the adoption and that she is not sure whether she is going to take their case. Visibly irked by the Lewins' attitude toward Khaila, she says that she understands why they chose a Black lawyer, but she lets them know what she thinks about their situation as a person of color. She believes that even if they raise a child "with the best intentions in the world, color-blind," "the world is still out there," and the child "needs to know who he is." She is framing the biological connection as integral to adequate nurture and, specifically, to cultural transfer. In response to Margaret's intense declaration—"A child should be with his parents"—she calmly states, "We agree there." This statement and Lewis's warning to Khaila leave ambiguous the decision of who should be a parent. The ambiguity points to the issues that arise when the culturally normative assumption of biocultural kinship as the context in which nature and nurture coincide is challenged by nontraditional kinship, which splits them and, in this case, challenges the correlation of kinship structures with the logic of the racial binary. Critics' and scholars' reactions to *Losing Isaiah* point to the default cultural understanding of this split as generating the need to make a choice. It is seen in the cultural response to the film's ending—a consistent rejection of its solution to the plot conflict.

The judge rules in Khaila's favor, but at the end of the film, Khaila calls Margaret because she cannot manage Isaiah's reaction to the loss of his adoptive family and because she recognizes Isaiah's suffering and knows what it feels like to be moved from one foster home to another. She wants Margaret to "hold him" until he "ain't scared no more." Khaila makes it clear that she is not giving up Isaiah again and that she is allowing Margaret to be present in his life when she explains, "I'm not saying I'm giving him back to you. I'm just saying he's going to come live with you for a little while till he can understand all this. Now, some people are going to think that I'm crazy, but I don't care. All that matters to me is Isaiah. And you may not like me, but you are going to have to deal with me." Margaret accepts this, and the two women symbolically confirm this new kinship bond by saying that they both love Isaiah and by hugging each other. It might look like Khaila is suggesting an open adoption in which a biological mother's contact with an adoptive family and child is mediated by an agreement that typically privileges permanency of adoptive bonds and limits biological parents' presence in a child's life. But in this case, it is Khaila who includes and determines the degree of Margaret's presence in the life of her son. Such family configuration does not comply with the model of parental exclusivity privileged in American culture, and it may have provoked misinterpretations of and negative responses to the film's ending, the meaning of which is difficult to pin down.

The conversation between Khaila and Margaret is followed by a scene that may have suggested to some viewers that the film's ending reverses the court's verdict and returns the child to Margaret. When she enters Isaiah's classroom,

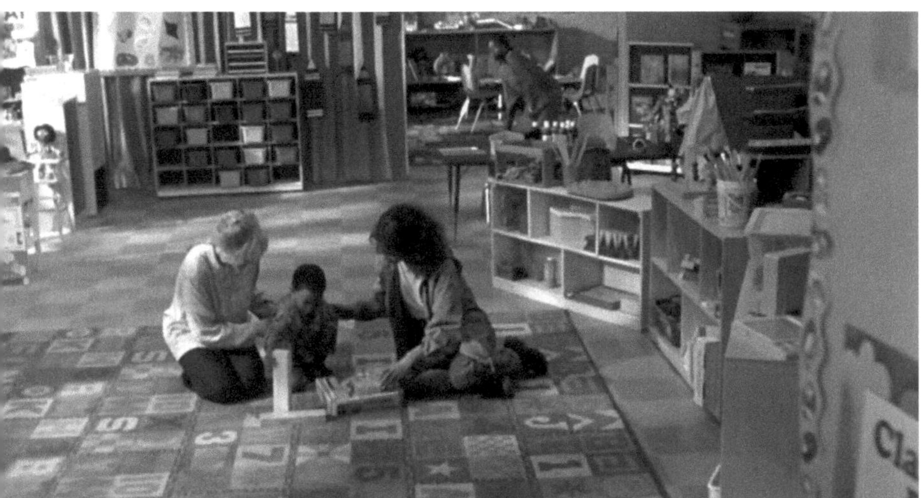

IGURE 1.2. The blocks play scene in *Losing Isaiah*. Paramount Pictures, 1995.

he rushes to her and calls her "mommy." The camera spins around Isaiah in Margaret's embrace, suggesting happy giddiness. At the same time, this camera movement is drawing a circle around the mother and child, enclosing them in their own space and leaving Khaila outside. But when the camera stops and frames Margaret, she says, "Thank you," and the camera cuts to Khaila's face—smiling through her tears and nodding lightly, happy with Isaiah's calming down. The delivery of Margaret's next line breaks the boundary around her and Isaiah and establishes her acknowledgment of Khaila. She asks Isaiah, "Can you show [pause] me and Khaila what you like to do?" The pause is emphasizing that she is deliberately including Khaila in their relationship with Isaiah, even though she is not calling her his mother. This scene can be read as continuing the theme of openness in adoption: the two women include each other in their relationship with Isaiah. Margaret's gesture is a response to Khaila's. But it may also be understood, by those who think that Isaiah is returned to Margaret permanently, as a reinstatement of the adoptive mother's control over the kinship structure. The concluding element of the reunion scene seems to clarify this ambiguity, as it shows how Isaiah himself envisions his family life. The women and Isaiah move to the rug in the middle of the room and play with blocks (see figure 1.2). Margaret asks him, "Is that a house? Which house is Khaila's house?" Isaiah replies, "This one, and this is yours," which suggests a separation of domestic spaces, none of which he calls his. But he places two blocks of equal height, representing the two houses, side by side, and Margaret calls it "Isaiah's tower" in which he can have a "room at the top." Isaiah's thinking about two domestic spaces in equal terms may indicate his refusal to make a choice between Khaila and Margaret, who both are going to be the foundation of his life. The cultural imperative to make a choice between mothers is neutralized by reimagining the solution to it as acceptance of all domestic spaces. The last image we see before the credits roll is two mothers—Black and white—playing with a Black child, sharing space on the same rug.

It is telling that more often than not, film critics and scholars either read the ending as the transfer of the child to Margaret or reject this solution to the plot conflict as implausible and unsatisfying. Susan Bordo, for example, writes that the film shows Khaila as "unable to comfort or care for [Isaiah]," so she "ultimately returns him to the social worker" (327). Daphne Wiggins considers "the finale . . . a fairy tale" (289). Wiggins sees the outcome of "Isaiah [living] happily ever after with two mothers, twice as much love, contact with his heritage in the African American community, and the amenities offered by his Caucasian family . . . [as] not realistic" (289–90). For Wiggins, a good outcome is "*a* willing, wanting family" (emphasis mine) that avails itself of the cultural knowledge necessary for Isaiah's identification and provides "the child [with] the best of both worlds in a stable environment" (290). Even though these two views of the ending differ, they share a common ground: neither imagines a child having two mothers. Similarly, film critics who see the film's conflict in binary terms have refused to see the unresolved binary choice of a mother as a plausible ending. Roger Ebert, who named the film's central questions as "Whom does the baby belong with? The parents it has bonded with? Or its biological mother?" called "the conclusion . . . a solution which, although it does allow the movie to end, really solves nothing" (1995). Desson Howe of *The Washington Post* saw the ending as a "a cop-out ending intended to offend no one and give everyone some note of satisfaction" in a "which-side-are-you-on? racial button pushing" situation. An overall more favorable review in *The New York Times* still pointed out "the impossibility of a viable ending to this story" and "no decent way out of this dilemma," which made the ending a "fake compromise" (Maslin). The refusal of the audiences to see the ending of *Losing Isaiah* as a satisfying closure points to a break in the genre logic that is supposed to happily "marry" historically specific cultural ideas about kinship and filmmaking conventions.

In family melodrama, where a painful separation of mother and child is central to the plot conflict, a happy ending depends on their reunion. Such an outcome is meant to evoke pleasure in the viewer given that the moral order has been restored. The adoption plot of *Losing Isaiah* leads to Isaiah's double reunion with the biological and adoptive mothers. Yet the viewers perceive this doubling of mothers not as doubly pleasurable but, instead, as a confusing failure to produce an acceptable family structure. Indeed, the reconciliatory sentiment of the final scene seems simplistic given the violent history of Black families' separation and the cultural climate around transracial adoption at the time. In this specific context, a rejection of nontraditional kinship that includes two mothers of different race and class points to the heterocoital family's role in maintaining hierarchical social divisions. The fact that the ending of *Losing Isaiah* does not ring true with the viewers points to the cultural distrust of the idea that kinship can suture social and cultural rifts by establishing kinship configurations that bring different races and classes together. This perceived "impossibility of a viable ending" (Maslin) in *Losing Isaiah* signals the incompatibility of culturally sanctioned kinds of relationships (inflected by race and class) and rules of child ownership (heterocoital trumps all) with the form of kinship Khaila and Margaret represent. It is worth noticing that both popular responses and more nuanced scholarly analyses of the film seem to share the expectation that a child needs *a* mother, not two.

"Monomaternalism," which Shelley Park defines as "an ideological doctrine" that "resides at the intersection of patriarchy . . . heteronormativity . . . capitalism . . . and Eurocentrism" and serves to erase diversity of kinship configurations, but primarily the possibility of several mothers for one child (7), is an idea that informs enduring cultural resistance to open adoptions, which has been observed by several scholars.[4] While various forms of open adoption had been practiced in the US prior to the postwar shift toward closed adoptions,[5] formalized open adoptions that included contact between adoptive and biological families were just beginning at the time of the film's release. According to Abbie E. Goldberg, the late 1980s and early 1990s "saw a marked shift in professional practices and attitudes," but the ideas about kinship associated with open adoptions did not take hold even within the professional community until the late 1990s (3). It is possible that

4. See Modell; Sales; Carp 2002a; Park. Shelley Park, specifically, unpacks the way in which monomaternalism works to maintain racial, class, and gender divisions through insisting on a single-mother kinship configuration.

5. The passing of "An Act to Provide for the Adoption of Children" in 1851 Massachusetts introduced the legal break between the child and the biological family, so that the adoptive family could be legally recognized as the child's only family (Carp 2002b, 6). It eventually became a model for other states. It paved the way to the philosophy of closed adoptions, initiated by the 1917 Children's Code of Minnesota, which "closed adoption records to public inspection" even though adoption triad members could see this information (Carp 2002b, 8). And closed adoptions became the rule after World War II. The difference between the open adoption of the post–closed adoption era versus informal open adoption is in the formal regulation of contact with adoptive and biological families.

the strong critical reaction to the ending of *Losing Isaiah* may be indicative of the contemporaneous cultural ideas about openness in adoption. But cultural resistance to open adoption practices does not seem to be a period-specific phenomenon. Several scholars point out that even as open adoption has become more widely practiced, the process and its impact on the participants remains largely misunderstood, and cultural resistance to open adoption is pervasive. Goldberg, for example, cites "even educated and worldly people" thinking that "a clean break would be better for everyone" because they imagine that having two families might be "confusing for the children," that birth parents might want to "move on and build a life for themselves," and that adoptive parents might feel "really jealous and upset" if the biological parents are present in the adopted child's life (1).

Even if open adoption is chosen by the parents, the way it is practiced reveals lingering nonacceptance of kinship structures that go beyond the nuclear biogenetic model. For example, Judith Modell's anthropological study of open adoption in the US found that this new way of kinship-making "does not create a new family or form new threads of kinship" (66). It only changes the way information about participants in adoption is circulated. Modell's criteria for kinship structure revisions include "diffuse and enduring solidarity" between the biological and adoptive parents who share a child (69). According to her, the intensity of private relationships between a child and parent figures may have the potential to change kinship and, perhaps, bridge some social divides, which, in turn, could lead to changes in the social fabric of society. However, open adoption in its current form fails to produce such relationships, since it does not even "meet cultural criteria for kinship" in many cases where the adoptive family's contact with biological parents is limited to correspondence (69). While it may seem like a paradox that cultural resistance to open adoption exists even as it is becoming more widely practiced, it may not be a paradox at all since cultural resistance to revisions of the nuclear biological family shape the practice of open adoption and produce kinship configurations that are nonthreatening to the heterocoital family and the social structures that it produces and supports. The availability of information about the adoptee's heterocoital origin takes care of the anxieties about the way the child was produced. And family belonging is still understood as secure if the nuclear heterocoital configuration (in the sense of having one set of parents of opposite sexes) is maintained, even if it is maintained through its imitation in adoption.

The larger culture may resist open adoption and other nontraditional kinship since it seems to be at odds with the culturally favored idea that "a nuclear family is best for a child" (Modell 63). Modell, however, puts such thinking in question by pointing out that the discussions of the child's best interest are concerned with "the integrity of the family" rather than "the person of the child" (191, 192). She demonstrates that the criteria for best interest "reflect and reinforce dominant social divisions and cultural values," which are heavily inflected by class and race in the US, and that the principle of the best interest of the child in adoption "naturalizes these interpretations by linking them to a child's well-being" (120, 192). Thus, the resistance to open adoption and other kinship structures that trouble the nuclear, biological model may be a rejection of affinities, affiliations, and identities that can grow across culturally determined social boundaries. The film's perceived failure to name only one woman Isaiah's mother indicates a rift between "the social and economic parameters surrounding child placement in the United States" and "the values that adoption historically upheld: family members should be alike; a child's interests are best served in a nuclear family; knowledge of her or his background is good for a child's 'adjustment'" (Modell 68, 70). In this light, *Losing Isaiah* is a negotiation of what families are possible in and acceptable to American society in terms of race, class, and repronormativity. Social disparities and misalignments along class and race lines complicate the decision about Isaiah's best interest, since it seems impossible to meet all the criteria by choosing only one mother. Neither Margaret nor Khaila is the "best mother" who fulfills all required conditions. The film does seem to position Khaila as such by showing her working hard to establish her new class standing, which earns her the viewer's respect and the custody of Isaiah. But just when she seems capable of giving her child both a sense of racial identity and a stable enough environment, the film complicates yet again the neat dichotomy of the "good" and "unfit" mothers produced by the ideology of placement by showing the traumatizing impact of the court's decision on the child.[6] While the narrative shows that it is the emotional separation that Isaiah is suffering from, the film also portrays Isaiah's new life as below the standard of living he used to enjoy with the Lewins. Khaila's small apartment with a dingy bathroom is no match for Margaret's house. When Isaiah is taken from Margaret, the social worker forbids him to bring his toys. It may be done to facilitate his "forgetting" of another family, but it also suggests that staying with his biological mother will mean living with more limited resources. This plot twist points to the inability of the social and legal structures that regulate kinship to fully solve pervasive systemic inequalities. It is then upon the two women to privately grapple with the consequences of inadequate welfare support for single

6. Meanwhile, Modell notes that "the majority of birthparents in the United States . . . share the characteristics of the presumptive adoptive family: middle class, white, and educated" (47–48).

mothers and the cultural, social, and legal rifts caused by racism. The judge's final verdict recognizes the "initial trauma" of Isaiah's separation from Margaret but says that Isaiah could overcome it if the adults "behave thoughtfully." It shifts the responsibility for Isaiah's well-being into the private space, leaving it to the adults in Isaiah's life to figure out what thoughtful behavior might be. But the move of the two mothers to solve the contradicting demands for the child's best interest by joining their care efforts is not accepted by the viewers as a believable outcome. In a culture committed to the nuclear biological family model that often serves to perpetuate social divisions, such kinship configuration may indeed look like a "fairy tale" (Wiggins 289). The audience's resistance to the ending's progressive vision of openness in adoption draws attention away from the fact that the underlying logic of the film still remains committed to the nuclear biological family model. Isaiah is ultimately given to Khaila, who does not intend to leave Isaiah with Margaret indefinitely. Margaret is remaining in his life to ease the emotional impact of the transition. She is saving the day, but her ability to envision Isaiah's long-term needs is discredited enough throughout the film to suggest that Isaiah, as Margaret's husband points out, would be "better off" with Khaila. Khaila is portrayed as ultimately possessing both the unconditional love grounded in a biological bond and a motherly affect that allows her to decide on care that is best for Isaiah. The cultural preference for the heterocoital family in which nature and nurture co-occur is thus reaffirmed, and, Isaiah's understanding of the situation notwithstanding, Margaret's parenting is defined by both Khaila and the court as temporary.

•

Over time, subtle changes in kinship ideas appear within mainstream adoption melodramas. A later, 2010 film *Mother and Child* presents a single Black mother as more acceptable to the larger culture, for example. *Mother and Child* also offers an interesting comparison point of the viewers' reactions, which reveals possible growing acceptance of nontraditional kinship configurations created through openness in adoption. The ending of *Mother and Child,* which will be discussed later in more detail, has not been criticized as much as *Losing Isaiah*'s, even though the ending has a scene visually and thematically similar to the last scene of *Losing Isaiah* (see figure 1.3).

Mother and Child weaves together stories of several women who have been touched by adoption in different ways. The film's narrative is framed by the story of Karen (Annette Bening). She became pregnant as a teenager and gave birth to her daughter at a home for pregnant young women. As a

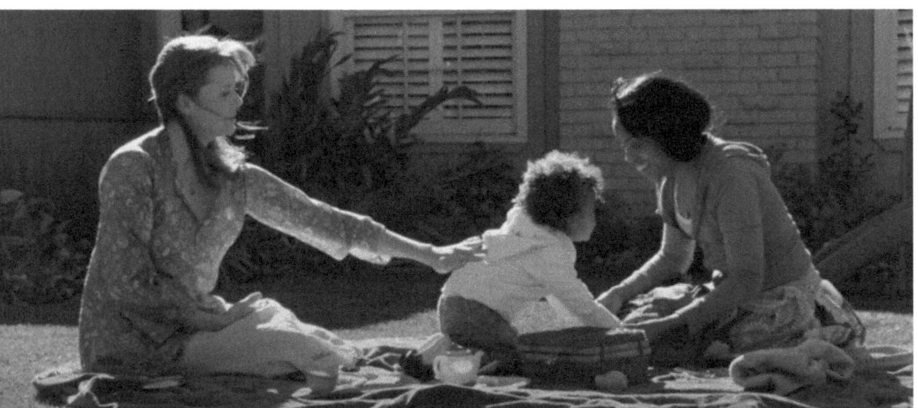

FIGURE 1.3. The blanket play scene in *Mother and Child.* Sony Pictures Classics, 2010.

legal guardian of her child, Karen's mother decided to relinquish the infant for adoption. The adoption was closed, as was common in the mid-twentieth century, so that the adoptive and the biological families would not have contact. Karen's storyline develops alongside those of two other women: Elizabeth (Naomi Watts), an adopted person who is eventually revealed to be Karen's biological daughter, and Lucy (Kerry Washington), a prospective adoptive mother. The film features one more mother—Ray (Shareeka Epps), who considers placing her child for adoption with Lucy but changes her mind. Karen and Elizabeth's storyline is structured around the tropes of the search and reunion plot, while Lucy and Ray are engaged in the birth-mother-as-a-threat drama. At the end of the film, these two storylines converge when Elizabeth's death during childbirth triggers a chain of events that leads to Lucy adopting Elizabeth's daughter and Karen getting a chance to meet this child, her granddaughter.

The action of the film starts after Karen and Elizabeth have been separated for thirty-seven years. Both women are presented as living in permanent emotional arrest, unable to develop deep relationships with people around them. Karen lives with her mother, who feels responsible for ruining Karen's life but does not talk about it openly with Karen. Their relationship is built on resentment and emotional distance. Karen cannot trust anyone. She is chronically suspicious of Sophia (Elpidia Carrillo), the caretaker who looks after Karen's ailing mother. She is jealous of her mother and Sophia's close relationship and of the connection Sophia has with her own daughter, Cristi. Karen's developing romance with Paco (Jimmy Smits) is punctuated by awkward moments and miscommunications due to her inability to open up emotionally. Elizabeth, too, avoids deep relationships. She is fiercely independent and is aggressively pursuing her career. She has chosen her own legal name—Elizabeth Joyce, and when she was seventeen, she had her tubes tied. Unwilling to maintain a stable relationship with anyone, she is also actively destroying relationships of others. We learn that she is not close to her adoptive mother, and her adoptive father died when she was young. She is angry at her biological mother and refuses to search for her.

Both Karen, a birth mother, and Elizabeth, an adopted person, are portrayed as traumatized by closed adoption. Both women have trouble experiencing and performing emotions of togetherness that are culturally central to kinship: openness, intimacy, and forgiveness. Such representations are in line with Katarina Wegar's (1996) observation that discourses around sealed birth records presume a difference of the adoption triad members from people related through traditional (a.k.a. biological) familial bonds. The lack of biological ties is represented in the film as an impediment to emotional expression that is culturally expected in the context of kinship. The film connects Karen's and Elizabeth's emotional deficits to their reproductive difference. This negative portrayal of adoption has not been lost on its reviewers. Peter Bradshaw from *The Guardian* called the film "oddly moralizing" and criticized its intolerance of "the idea that one woman could give up a child to another for adoption, and that all concerned could live with this arrangement reasonably happily." O. A. Scott from *The New York Times* wrote that the film was portraying adoption as "something close to a catastrophe, a tear in the fabric of the natural order," and wondered if such stance "may baffle or alienate viewers whose experience suggests otherwise." Such reviews critique what they perceive to be a monolithic narrative of adoption as a traumatizing, unnatural practice. But the film does portray an outcome of adoption that the viewer is expected to experience as a happy ending. It is Lucy's adoption of Ella, Elizabeth's biological daughter. Rather than offering a blanket portrayal of adoption as a cause of injurious difference, *Mother and Child*'s affective arc takes the viewer from sadness about Elizabeth's and Karen's losses associated with closed adoption toward a feeling of redemption that accompanies a recovery and preservation of biological ties through openness in adoption process.

Karen and Elizabeth experience an emotional awakening as a result of a reestablished biological connection between a mother and her biological child. Elizabeth changes emotionally after discovering her impossible pregnancy. She quits her demanding job as a partner in a law firm, breaks off her affair with her boss, Paul (Samuel L. Jackson), who is the father of the child, and comes to terms with becoming a mother. She insists on delivering the baby naturally, so she can see her and bond with her—the opposite of what may have happened to her own biological mother (it was not uncommon at the time to take the newborn away without so much as letting the woman see it). The prospect of becoming a mother by birth changes her mind about meeting her own biological mother. She writes a letter expressing her wish to receive communications from her and leaves it with the adoption agency, which can bring them together if Karen decides to search for Elizabeth too—under the conditions of their adoption, the agency can only reveal information if both parties agree to it. Karen's awakening begins with an indirect apology she receives after her mother's death when Sophie reveals that Karen's mother felt responsible for ruining her daughter's life. Karen is freed by this recognition of her suffering and the non-normalcy of closed adoption arrangement. Gradually, she learns to trust others enough to marry Paco and consider searching for Elizabeth. She writes a letter expressing this intent and waits for Elizabeth to do the same. Due to a clerical error—Elizabeth's letter is misplaced—Karen cannot reunite with Elizabeth in time. Elizabeth dies in childbirth, and her daughter is adopted by Lucy. When Karen finds out that Elizabeth is dead, she is distraught and resentful of Paco, who encouraged her to look. She thinks that Elizabeth could have still been alive to her if she did not know of her death. Perhaps, comparing this situation to her own, she seems to think that her connection to Elizabeth is over, since the baby has been given up for adoption. To her, adoption means a closed adoption with slim chance of contact. But the film ends with Karen's emotional healing after she gets Lucy's permission to meet Ella, her biological granddaughter. Ella's adoption is facilitated by the same adoption agency that handled Karen's case, which underscores the change that has happened in adoption practice. Karen's visit with Lucy and Ella is arranged by the same nun (Cherry Jones) who facilitated both Karen's search for Elizabeth and Lucy's adoption attempts.

When Karen receives the address, she starts laughing uncontrollably. The next cut explains why. We see Karen walking out of her house and going just to the end of the block: Lucy and Ella live in the same neighborhood. Karen is walking slowly. The day is windy—it suggests change and Karen's emotional turmoil. The camera is trained on Karen's apprehensive face; she seems unsure about what she is doing until she walks past the camera and the angle changes as if suggesting that Karen has decided to keep going. As Karen approaches Lucy's house, we see Lucy and Ella lounging on a blanket on their lawn. They are bathed in soft sunlight, and the wind now gives the scene an air of lightness. Lucy rises as Karen comes up; they smile at each other, and then we see the two women playing peekaboo with Ella. Ella is running circles around the blanket where Karen and Lucy sit, enclosing them as if she is holding them together—an echo of the visual language used in the last scene of *Losing*

Isaiah to suggest a new, expanded kinship boundary. The endings of both films feature two women, Black and white, playing with a child. Both scenes are suggestive of open adoption and kinship across race lines. But the critical response has been much more accepting of openness in adoption as plot resolution in *Mother and Child.* The ending of *Mother and Child* has not been met with the degree of misunderstanding and nonacceptance seen in reactions to the ending of *Losing Isaiah.* In fact, it was hardly mentioned in any of the reviews.

It may be tempting to read the ending, and the viewers' acceptance of it, as evidence of changes in cultural attitudes to open adoption that crosses race lines. The emotional arc of the narrative is moving the viewer from manifestations of arrested mother-child affect toward its free-flowing expression in the scene on the blanket. This emotional script draws attention to the difference between the traumatic outcomes of closed adoption and the healing that open adoption may provide. The happy reunion scene places Black and white bodies next to each other, and the emotional charge of the scene suggests mutual acceptance and reconciliation. Ella, a child of a white mother and a Black father, is cared for by her Black adoptive mother and a white grandmother. It is worth noticing, though, some differences between the endings of *Losing Isaiah* and *Mother and Child* that may have reduced the anxiety of the viewer about the kinship arrangement in the latter. The emotional impact of this scene on the viewer is carefully modulated. Ella's tie to her biological mother is deactivated through Elizabeth's death, while her connection to her biological origin, which open adoption is supposed to maintain, is weakly acknowledged through the presence of her biological grandmother. In a culture where the normative heterocoital family structure functions to separate races, racial matching of the child and her adoptive mother simultaneously weakens Ella's tie to the biological mother and strengthens the imitation of a heterocoital tie to the adoptive family. In this way, the film manages to avoid the two-mothers dilemma while still underscoring the power of heterocoital family ties (i.e., blood ties) to heal all parties to adoption. The possibility of adoption disruption by biological relatives is diminished since there is no definitive decision in the film that Ella's is going to be an open adoption. Even though Karen is Ella's biological family, she is warned by the nun who oversees adoption services that she has no legal claim to the child because Elizabeth was not legally her daughter, and it would be "up to the mother"—Lucy—whether the child knows who Karen is. The film is ambiguous about whether this will happen. The nonthreatening character of this arrangement is emphasized by its contrast with Lucy and Ray's narrative line, which demonstrates the power of an active biological connection between a mother and a child to jeopardize an adoption. Ray withdraws her consent to transfer her newborn to Lucy after she delivers the baby, and Lucy experiences a breakdown. The fact that in *Mother and Child* the adoptive mother and child's bond is secured by the death of the birth mother suggests that kinship negotiations in the film are not a matter of an argument about closed versus open adoption. It is, rather, a matter of negotiating nontraditional kinship in a way that leaves heterocoital ideology in place. A child can still have just one mother.

Mother and Child does not ask the question "Who is the mother?" or "What makes the mother?" It conveniently does away with ambivalences about these questions by removing excess mothers in the kinship configurations portrayed in the film. Elizabeth's adoptive family is erased from the narrative save for a brief explanation Elizabeth gives to Paul. We only follow the storyline that connects her to her biological mother, Karen. Ray's storyline reinforces the cultural primacy of the biological bond. Elizabeth dies. Karen's story does not end with the scene on the blanket. She comes home after and tells Paco, "She has my mother's eyes," using physical resemblance to establish genetic continuity that ties four women in her bloodline together. That night she addresses Elizabeth in her diary and writes that she has accepted never having known Elizabeth, and that the "horrible parade" of thirty-eight years they were apart is now "past," because "Ella is peace." The film ends with Karen in bed, turned away from Paco toward the nightstand on which she has arranged pictures of pregnant Elizabeth and her biological father as a fourteen-year-old boy. Ella, a body that is racially different from the people in the photos, is in the picture without appearing in it. Karen falls asleep looking at them, comforted by a "restored" heterocoital family that, incidentally, remains racially homogenous in its presentation.[7]

By manipulating spatial arrangement of Black and white, biologically related and adoptive bodies, the film manages to simultaneously affirm biological and adoptive families as long as they are in line with the heterocoital model. This modulation makes evident the power of the heterocoital model to inscribe other forms of difference: race, in this case. The culturally imperative need for a known biological (heterocoital) origin, which is foundational to open adoption practices, is satisfied safely in an adoptive family as long as the other mother is bracketed out of a family configuration, as it is for Lucy. The other mother's significance can also be downplayed, as happens with the adopted persons in the film (Elizabeth and Ella) or when the situation of uncertain child ownership is disambiguated and the biological connection

7. Heterocoital reproduction is reaffirmed in yet another scene: after her own mother's death, Karen makes contact and sleeps with the Elizabeth's biological father, as if trying to enact what her mother forbade her and to revive the heterocoital connection to her lost daughter.

is fully reinstated, as illustrated by the character Ray. In Lucy's case, the use of race as a stand-in for blood and biological connection legitimizes Lucy's adoptive family as a successful imitation of the heterocoital one. It reduces the complexity of Ella's biological origin by shifting focus off her being biracial, and such visual erasure of possible "diffuse and enduring solidarity" between the biological and adoptive parents (Modell 69) reinforces heterocoital kinship's power to keep social divisions in place.

This ultimate reinscription of divisions seems to be at odds with the ethos of *Mother and Child*'s subgenre—the fragmented narrative that critics and scholars have called the "hyperlink movie" (Ebert 2005), "fractal" (Everett), "ensemble" (Hsu), or "network cinema" (Silvey). Broadly speaking, these terms describe films that feature separate storylines of different characters that converge by the end of the film and make sense as elements of a single event or narrative that binds them together. The viewer's understanding of characters and their motivations grows and changes in the light of progressively exposed connections. Vivien Silvey calls network cinema a "genre [that] belongs to a broader contemporary imaginary concerning social networks" (583) and points to the genre's emergence as a response to social disruptions caused by technology and globalization. Understood as such, network film is seen as "re-imagin[ing] pluralistically societies and communities that are usually conveyed as distinct and separate" (Silvey 585). The anxiety about alienation and miscommunication potentially caused by such pluralism is met by narrative strategies that lead "the viewer . . . to conceive of the characters as a cosmopolitan community," as connected in spite of a lack of "spatial, familial, cultural and racial bounds" (583). Such ethos of network cinema maps well onto the logic of melodramatic imagination, which Brooks describes as a reaction to "a frightening new world in which the traditional patterns of moral order no longer provide the necessary social glue" (20). In the absence of certainty about the moral order, Brooks says, melodrama reestablishes the "moral universe" (20). As a network melodrama, *Mother and Child* responds to cultural anxieties about nontraditional kinship: adoption, single motherhood, and racially diverse biological families. Offering its vision of strangers serendipitously connected by biological kinship as a remedy for genealogical uncertainties, the film reinstates biological kinship and origin as the "necessary social glue" (20) that heals one's sense of self and keeps communities together, even though the plot of the film seems to suggest a more open idea of kinship that can cross the boundaries biogenetic kinship typically serves to maintain.

As *Mother and Child* demonstrates, in adoption melodrama, negotiations may be quite complex between "old" and "new" forms of experience, resulting in a reestablishment of "the existence of a moral universe" against the obstacles mounted by "perversions of judgment" (Brooks 20). Gledhill and Williams (2018) claim that the logic of reestablishing the moral order involves potential mismatching of lived experiences with the ones that are recognized culturally and legally and that conform to the contemporaneous structures of feeling. According to Gledhill, "if melodramatic modality aims to render everyday life morally legible . . . it must, in order to command recognition, acknowledge the contested and changing signs of cultural verisimilitude, bringing radical as well as conservative voices into play" (2000, 236). The presence of such tensions in melodramatic narratives doesn't mean that the moral order is necessarily reinvented. Even though *Mother and Child* portrays an acceptance of kinship forms that depart from the nuclear biological model, it solicits such acceptance from the viewer by still linking kinship to heterocoital reproduction and knowledge of biological origin, imagined as permanent bonds that hold communities together. Openness in adoption does not serve, in the end, the project of expanding the nuclear family configuration. Even though in the film, family separation and community dissolution are explicitly associated with closed adoption that helps imitation of the heterocoital family, threats that open adoption presents to such family are still alleviated through imagining kinship on the terms set by the heterocoital framework.

The return to familiar ideas about heterocoital reproduction and kinship as a response to anxiety about social cohesion is a recognizable move that has been used toward a variety of political ends. In response to the social threat of the new freedoms that individuals can experience in nontraditional kinship relationships, a return to traditional family values is invoked as a way to hold communities together across generations. For example, citing "policing of mothers" in Black and Native American communities in *Somebody's Children,* Laura Briggs shows that social anxieties about cultural challenges to nuclear family, reproduction, and heteronormativity have been stoked as pretexts for "the reorganization of race, the state, and economic resources" to preserve the white heteropatriarchal status quo (9). While it may seem that the end of the twentieth and the beginning of the twenty-first centuries have been an era of "choice in relationships" and friendship as the new emerging social glue (Chambers 1), adoption scholars, who have been engaging with the social significance of both social and biological ties, insist on the growing cultural importance of "'blood' kin, especially ascendant and descendant kin," in cultures where "marriage and other heterosexual pair-bonding becomes less secure" (Norval, qtd. in Wegar 120).[8] Adoption is the context that fore-

8. Also see Briggs; Latchford on cultural primacy of the biogenetic family.

shadows what might be in store when heterocoital origin and the universality of the heterocoital parent-child bond are destabilized by new technologies of reproduction and kinship that lead to new ways of social life. Cinematic portrayals of adoption corroborate what Franklin and McKinnon (2001) have already suggested in their studies of new forms of kinship: when traditional reproduction can no longer reliably underpin social structures reliant on heterocoital order, heterocoital family still survives as a metaphor that structures other kinds of kinship and social ties.

Adoption melodrama develops such a metaphorical apparatus, as it addresses anxieties about nontraditional kinship and reinstates the idea of heterocoital origin as an anchor of human identity, and the heterocoital family model, even in its imitative expression, as a site of personal and social stability. It assures, in Brooks's words, the inevitable triumph of reproductive "virtue" over "villainy" and "demonstrates over and over that the sign of ethical forces can be discovered and can be made legible" (20). ARTs dramas show, too, that while lived experiences may be reaching beyond a family in which nature and nurture co-occur, toward a world where nature and nurture can be split between parents and genitors, biogenetic-assumed-heterocoital origin remains a constant, a cultural imperative, and a universal human identity anchor. In its metaphorical iteration, it also remains the nontraditional kinship anchor: a nontraditional family is culturally acceptable, albeit still different and subjected to normalizing discourses, if a child's biogenetic origin is known, assumed, or imagined as heterocoital. Above all, heterocoital origin remains an anchor to heteronormativity: adoption and ARTs are predominantly narrated and understood through heterocoital metaphors as imitations of a heterocoital family and heterocoital heteronormative reproduction. As long as non-heterocoital family can be imagined as heterocoital, everything is all right.

This idea informs *The Kids Are All Right* (2010) by Lisa Cholodenko, one of the few mainstream films that portray ARTs and same-sex families. It responds to the growing visibility of same-sex marriages and aims to normalize a two-mother family by portraying a lesbian couple, Nic (Annette Bening) and Jules (Julianne Moore), engaged in typical middle-class suburban family life. The film was well received by the majority of viewers, who saw it as "the best movie about lesbians" (Dolan) or "a film about marriage itself, an institution with challenges that are universal" (Ebert 2010). Yet, it was critiqued by the opponents of gay marriage, who typically found it too homonormative.[9] Such cultural response makes sense given the logic of kinship representation

9. See scholarship by Duggan; Eaklor, etc. for a discussion of this perspective.

in the film: queer marriage and family life are represented through familiar heteronormative tropes. The film's portrayal of a lesbian reproductive family as a simulacrum of heteronormative, heterocoital kinship provides a nonthreatening way of thinking about a two-mother family.

The clearly gendered roles of each mother in the relationship make this family more palatable to the viewers invested in the heterocoital family model. Nic is obviously the head of the household, its primary breadwinner. She is controlling and direct; her drinking problem is the way she copes with emotional turmoil. Jules is a gentler, more emotionally open, stay-at-home mother. She is trying to start her own business after the children have grown up, and she needs a lot of reassurance, which Nic often fails to give. The gendered characteristics are so obviously polarized that when Jules says to Nic: "You have always wanted a wife!" it does not come as a surprise to the viewer. Since "two mothers can only squeeze into genealogical templates if there are no fathers" (Patton-Imani 15), this family is normalized for the viewer by reassigning the gender "missing" from the couple to Nic. The family configuration—children living with two married mothers—is obviously nontraditional. But there is no ambiguity about the reproductive process that made this family possible. Nic and Jules each gave birth to their own biological child—Joni (Mia Wasikowska) and Laser (Josh Hutcherson) respectively—with the sperm from the same donor. "Sharing" the donor material creates a connection that binds the family together, a genetic tie between the children, who are "real," a.k.a. genetic, siblings. The donor's biological material also links the two mothers in a way that approaches the heterocoital. The origin and identity of each child as well as the origin of the family are anchored in the as-if heterocoital narrative, in which everyone is connected through the genetic material of a single man. This plot move is a version of cultural "normalization of IVF" through its absorption into "the structure of bilateral, biological kinship norms" (Franklin 6–7). In *Biological Relatives,* Sarah Franklin draws attention to the "curious" logic of the cultural imagination around IVF, which on the one hand has become "routine" and naturalized through the familiar "sexual, gender, and kinship norms," but on the other hand has remained "a confusing and stressful world of disjointed temporalities, jangled emotions, difficult decisions, unfamiliar procedures, medical jargon, and metabolic chaos" (6–7). *The Kids Are Alright* eschews the portrayal of strangeness in the reproductive process and presents its successful result: a family created through ART. Its narrative conflicts are focused on cultural anxieties about this resulting family that represents "'marrying up' a biological model of sexual reproduction with a biologically based system of descent and family formation" (Franklin 6).

In its exploration of an as-if heterocoital queer family that visibly undermines cultural assumptions about reproduction and kinship, the film addresses cultural fears around the potential of ARTs to separate reproduction from heteronormativity. Its melodramatic imagination is working out a moral order that can respond to the threats posed by non-heterocoital families to heteropatriarchy. By the heteronormative logic, ARTs introduce the splitting of the imitated heterocoital reproduction from its culturally "real" version, or, as Franklin points out, "this marriage of cells now exists in two forms as a result of IVF—the one occurring in vivo, and the other in glass" (6). Such modification to heterocoital reproduction needs to be acculturated if heteronormativity and heterocoital order are to be preserved. Typically, Western cultures handle it by extending heteronormativity and gender beyond the hetero coitus onto the fusion of the biological material from genitors in a petri dish, outside of the bodies participating in reproduction.[10] The plot of *The Kids Are Alright,* similar to adoption search and reunion narratives, resolves the tension between what is considered culturally "real" and what is "as-if" by examining how Joni and Laser's reunion with their biological father-donor impacts their family. The central conflict of *The Kids Are Alright* is the threat to a nuclear family's integrity posed by children looking to engage with the man behind the biological material that has been their known point of origin. As in adoption search and reunion narratives, the children have to negotiate their difference from the culturally normative identity, and the family structure is challenged to accommodate kinship excess, but the questions raised by the film suggest a different way of looking at the need to know one's heterocoital origin and the way to deal with the doubling of mothers.

Laser and Joni's motivation for connecting with the biological father is somewhat different from the typical search and reunion narrative's motivation to know one's origin. The film keeps our knowledge of each child's as-if heterocoital origin activated. The children know how they were conceived and can access the information about their donor after turning eighteen. They live with their biological mothers, and the genetic continuity between mothers and children is emphasized by the likeness of their personalities. Joni is driven, or rather pushed, by professionally successful Nic to excel in academics. It becomes apparent in family arguments that Joni's successes are a way for Nic to prove the normalcy of a two-mother family. It is not accidental that a more "masculine" mother is concerned with showing that a nontraditional family can raise well-adjusted children. Laser, like his biological mother, Jules,

10. As Emily Martin has shown, the gendering of egg and sperm has been happening in science already, so this leap is not unexpected. The issue described by Martin has remained persistent.

is less sure of who he is and what he wants to do. In fact, it is through these two characters that the film's underlying question—are the kids alright without a man in the family?—is introduced.

The film starts with Laser's quest for masculinity in the absence of a male parent. The opening sequence tracks Laser and his friend Clay riding their bikes "like bats out of hell" to Clay's house (*The Kids Are Alright* 2010a).[11] The rough energy suggested by the cuts and the soundtrack signals Laser's search for expressions of masculinity less refined and more physical than Nic's. His looking for such male presence is obvious when he is watching with "a trace of longing" his friend's roughhousing with his dad (*The Kids Are Alright* 2010a). The film suggests that this longing is the reason why Laser convinces his reluctant sister, who is already eighteen and therefore can initiate a search and contact with their donor, to find their biological father. The question of whether the kids—and the family—can be alright without a male father becomes more complex after donor Paul (Mark Ruffalo) is brought into the family's life. The obvious quasihetero gendering of mothers has already stabilized the family as a successful imitation of a heterocoital one, and, before Paul appears, the family seems complete. For all its nontraditional same-sex parenting makeup, it remains in the heteronormative and heterocoital territory. Nic fulfills the fathering role, and the sperm from Paul anchors the children's knowledge of their as-if heterocoital origin; both children have a biological connection to the parents that are raising them. Yet Paul is still sought out and engaged by Laser and Joni, and his presence introduces a disruption into the stabilized nuclear family of Nic and Jules. The melodramatic arc that negotiates between the imitation of the heterocoital and the possibility to restore a full biological heterocoital configuration is reminiscent of the concerns typical of adoption search and reunion plots, but the "competition" of kin is reimagined. While adoption narratives often revolve around a choice between two mothers, in *The Kids Are Alright* the two-mother anxiety is recast as a choice between two fathers (who are often absent or neglected in adoption plots). The logic of the film's narrative seems to pit Paul, the biological father, against Nic, who is the social "father" in her family. The film thus invites us to consider the meaning of the father in the "moral order" (Brooks 20) of kinship by presenting Paul as seemingly unnecessary yet needed by the children.

With the introduction of Paul, the normalized queer family is re-queered, and the viewer is invited to consider whether and on what condition the culture can accept a family whose configuration is in excess of the

11. Note that the screenplay for *The Kids Are Alright,* written by Cholodenko and Stuart Blumberg, is also analyzed here and is cited as *The Kids Are Alright* 2010a. The film itself, directed by Cholodenko, is cited as *The Kids Are Alright* 2010b.

heteronormative, nuclear model. Like an adoptive family configuration, this one challenges the assumed continuity of nature and nurture in traditional kinship, but the nature-nurture split is complicated further. *The Kids Are Alright* takes us beyond the usual dualistic alignments of nature with biological parents (often mothers) and culture/nurture with nonbiological parents and fathers, whose role in child upbringing is often understood as social. Nic is the social father of the family, yet she is simultaneously a biological mother to one of the children. While an adoption search and reunion narrative is concerned with a binary choice between nature and nurture (often represented by the biological and the adoptive mothers) that has to be handled dialectically in a way that reaffirms both the importance of heterocoital origin and the "realness" of the adoptive family, the choices in *The Kids Are Alright* are not so binary. Thinking about the meaning of the father trifurcates the split between the "real" and the "as-if" into (1) nature as as-if heterocoital but genetically real connection (due to Paul's donated sperm and Nic and Jules being biological mothers); (2) nurture as a social function of fatherhood (Nic's or Paul's); and—in addition to the familiar binary—we are invited to consider the importance of (3) the embodied male and masculine presence of the father (Paul). The first two elements are present in Nic and Jules's family, and they serve to stabilize its nonnormative configuration by approximating the heterocoital, but why might Paul's adult parental male body be needed in this family?

It does not seem accidental that the question about this need arises in the context of a lesbian family. Paul's presence might be a response to the threat same-sex reproduction poses to heterocoital reproduction, heteronormativity, and patriarchy itself. The structure of the film suggests that the negotiation of his belonging in the family may be a negotiation of the cultural anxiety about the sexuality of a child brought up in a same-sex family. The opening sequence that typically frames films' main concerns draws attention to Laser's and Joni's sexualities. The first three scenes of the film intercut between Laser hanging out with Clay and Joni playing scrabble with her best girl friend, Sasha, and her best guy friend, Jai. On the first viewing of the film and in the absence of its larger context, Laser's fascination with male physical contact—he wrestles with Clay and "longingly" observes Clay's wrestling with his dad—may suggest a reading of his sexuality as at least ambivalent. Joni is taunted by Sasha to enjoy "some hot jock sausage" in college or at least admit that Jai and Joni have a crush on each other and "just do it." Joni and Jai "blush" and dodge this conversation. While their relationship is more suggestive of heterosexuality, Joni's uncertainty and reticence around it introduce enough ambiguity to raise questions about her sexuality when the three opening scenes cut to the family dinner and the viewer understands that Laser and Joni have been raised by a same-sex couple.

In response to fraught moments like this, Paul's heterosexual presence is often summoned to alleviate the viewers' anxieties about challenges to heterocoital reproduction and familiar expressions of (especially masculine) sexuality. For example, Paul's receiving the news that children conceived with his sperm are looking for him is followed by him and Tanya, a waitress in his restaurant, enjoying "a hot, sweaty fuck" (*The Kids Are Alright* 2010a). The strangeness of artificial conception and the relationships it produces is offset by a "natural" heterosexual act. In another example, a tension built through a sequence of queer events is resolved the moment Paul is mentioned. The sequence begins with Joni looking up the cryobank phone number that will help her and Laser locate their biological father at the same time as Nic and Jules are trying to have sex while watching male gay porn. Their choice of viewing material challenges and complicates the viewers' thinking about their sexualities, as it does about Laser's after he and Clay find the tape in his mothers' bedroom while looking for weed. Clay and Laser are "caught" watching the tape by Jules, and during the "talk" between Laser and the two moms, he expresses his confusion—should not they want to watch two women having sex? This discussion of complexities in human sexuality is tabled because Nic and Jules pursue their own, more straightforward questions in this conversation. They want to know if Laser and Clay "are fucking." Gay porn–watching seems to confirm what Nic and Jules have suspected, and they are concerned not so much about Laser's sexual orientation as about his choice of partner. Nic does not want Laser "exploring with that loser" Clay, and she wants Laser to come out to them, so she can make it known what is acceptable in this situation. But Laser mistakenly interprets "Are you having a relationship with someone?" as a question about his secret meeting with Paul, and the ensuing conversation, where he and his moms are talking at cross-purposes, ratchets up the mothers' and the viewers' anxiety about certain expressions of gay male sexuality. While Laser is talking about Paul, whom he only met once and with Joni's help, Nic and Jules suspect that Laser is talking about a weird "setup" of an encounter with a risky gay partner. The viewers are privy to the misunderstanding, and for them the conversation that invokes clichéd fears of dangerous, random, and exploitative gay sexuality is supposed to represent a moment of comic relief. The intended humor of the scene at once acknowledges and dismisses the fears. The resolution to the misunderstanding—Laser tells his moms about Paul and exclaims, "Wait! Did you guys think I was gay?!"—shows that he "is alright." The comedic buildup of cultural fears about wild homosexuality, which culminates in Laser's affirmation of his heterosexuality, neutralizes the imagined threat of the same-sex family to the heteronormative order. It is not accidental that information about Paul is instrumental to this resolution.

The talk about Laser's suspected homosexuality ends with an affirmation of Laser's heterosexuality when Paul becomes the subject of the conversation. Structurally, it looks like heterosexuality, represented by Paul in the film, frames the expressions of nonnormative sexuality and repeatedly "brings us back" from the brink of the imagined collapse of the heteronormative moral order and its homonormative variations in the film. The scene of Clay and Laser finding porn is, in fact, framed with scenes involving Paul, whose heterosexuality is on display from the moment he is introduced. For example, he is shown smiling at the "nasty talk" of Brooke, another waitress at his restaurant, while he is having lunch with Tanya. This scene cuts in between the scene of Nic and Jules wondering if Laser is gay and the one of the boys rummaging through Jules and Nic's drawers. The anxiety about Joni's sexuality is also resolved with Paul haunting the scene. She tries to kiss Jai after hanging out with Sasha, who keeps going on about Paul's sexual attractiveness: "Spermster's a hottie. Is he single?" The question implicit in the film's title is thus specified further: "Are kids' sexualities going to be alright in the absence of heterosexual role modeling in the family?" And the answer is: they are, because Paul's heterosexual male presence infuses heterosexuality into the family.

But Paul becomes a threat to the family's homonormative integrity after Paul has sex with Jules. This postconception coitus creates a possibility of a more "real" heterocoital family configuration that could normalize a part of the family further via post-factum naturalization of its reproduction. The emotional landscape of the film, however, invites the viewer to reject this possibility in favor of restoring the homonormative family of Nic and Jules. After the truth of Jules and Paul's affair comes out, Paul suggests they "get the kids together and do this thing," but he is rejected by Jules, who reminds him, "Jesus, Paul! I'm gay!" Several interactions with the family members show that Paul's understanding of the situation is off, likely because he perceives it as a typical heterosexual love-triangle conflict. His suggestion shows that he interprets Jules's behavior narrowly within the heterosexual/homosexual binary, and he is overlooking the significance of Joni's biological connection to Nic, who is not just a "father" of the family but also a biological mother to Joni. This complexity highlights the difference between the ways ART and adoptive families negotiate their belonging in heterocoital cultures. In her analysis of lesbian kinship, Sandra Patton-Imani observes the spilling of the adoption vocabulary into the same-sex family context. Specifically, she notices the distinction between biological and nonbiological mothers made through the use of the term "birth mother" to describe the partner who gave birth to a child. But the "birth mother" in same-sex families is not the vanished biological mother of an adoptee. The term is used to designate the culturally "real" mother and to anchor the biological bond and the origin of the child. Legally, the distinction between same-sex parents is preserved in the term "second parent," used in the case of secondary adoption by a nonbiological mother (17). *The Kids Are Alright* presents a scenario where each mother is a "birth mother" to her own child, and by sharing the sperm donor, they have created an as-if heterocoital connection between themselves and children. This configuration puts them on a more or less equal footing. The problem of two mothers is resolved by gendering the parental roles of Nic and Jules. Post-conception heterocoitus, however, gives more cultural value to Paul, Jules, and Laser's "side of the family" and suggests a hierarchy of parents based on the *kind* of biological connection (a biological mother is more important than a biological father, and both are more important than the "second parent"). When Nic reproaches Jules for "work[ing] out [her] issues by fucking other people," Jules says that Paul is "not just 'other people!'" perhaps suggesting a certain intimacy that may justify her behavior. Nic responds, also recognizing the connection between them and the donor as special, "No, you had to go fuck our sperm donor! You couldn't have picked a more painful way to hurt me" (*The Kids Are Alright* 2010a). The way Nic phrases her injury as "more hurtful" with a "sperm donor" suggests that she is not just upset that Jules has had sex with someone else or that she has had it with a man. The betrayal she experiences is reproductive, not sexual. In her conflict with the biological father of the children, Nic is thus doubly threatened. She is afraid she is going to be displaced in her paternal role by Paul because the as-if heterocoital family only has room for one, and Paul is biogenetically connected to the children. But the family does not have room for two mothers either. Hetero sex between Jules and Paul derealizes Nic's connection to Laser by making the fact that she is just the second parent to him obvious, and it also puts her connection with Joni in jeopardy even though she is Joni's biological mother. The hard won as-ifness of Nic and Jules's family is threatened by a multiplication of parents caused by the non-heterocoital conception.

The family that survives in the film is the family that can have just one father and one mother. When Paul stops by hoping for a reconciliation with Joni before she leaves for college, Nic confronts him and says, "This is not your family. This is my family! You're just a fucking interloper. . . . If you want a family so much, go out and make one of your own!" Nic claims the ownership of her family in a very masculine way by asserting its monogamy, and this confrontation seems like a dispute between two men or two fathers. But at this moment of establishing which family is "real" within the moral order of melodramatic imagination, her being a biological mother strengthens her claim. Nic wins, and Paul's wrong take on the situation is emphasized by the family's solidarity in expelling him from their circle: he is shown literally outside the family home, looking in through the window but ignored. The ending restores the monogamous nuclear family configuration, in which the responsibility for the children is clearly assigned to two parents who fulfill gendered paternal and maternal roles. The final scenes suggest the feeling of restored happiness by showing the moms and children locked in a group hug as they say goodbye to Joni on college campus. Later, as the moms and Laser are driving home, a close-up of Jules's hand touching Nic's knee and Nic holding Jules's hand signals that the parents have reconnected. Laser sees it and smiles too, "grateful for a sign" (*The Kids Are Alright* 2010a).

Nic's victory in recovering her family and the family's reconciliation suggest that the film's moral universe is open to the idea of nontraditional kinship formations. The happy ending does reject the possibility of Paul and Jules's heteronormative family since Paul is put outside the family circle as soon as he tries to make the family both heterocoital and heteronormative. And the film does gesture toward the possibility of expanding the idea of acceptable nontraditional kinship further by showing three biological parents and children getting along in a scene that features a dinner party at Paul's house. But this acceptance is short-lived because Nic discovers evidence of Jules's infidelity immediately after the "happy family" mise-en-scène is established (*The Kids Are Alright* 2010a). The ending's reinstatement of the homonormative lesbian reproductive family is not challenged enough to claim that this family configuration goes beyond as-if heterocoital; its ties to heteronormativity are preserved. A family with two lesbian biological mothers and a biological father who has had sex with one of them seems too much to bear for heteronormative cultural scripts that work to maintain the link between heterosexuality and heterocoital reproduction as a condition for the reproduction of heteronormative, heterocoital, patriarchal culture.

The film's ending invites the viewer to experience satisfaction with the restored monogamous nuclear family configuration. Even though Paul is expelled from the family, his embodied presence, beyond his genetic material, has naturalized IVF. His initially unbridled heterosexuality is disciplined through his contact with homonormative Nic and Jules, and this affirms the social value of the homonormative monogamous family. His desire to leave behind engagements with several women and create a family with Jules shows what the nuclear, heterocoital, reproductive family is for—channeling sexuality into socially acceptable forms that perpetuate heteronormativity and reproductivity. Ultimately, *The Kids Are Alright* shows that a family need not be heterosexual to reproduce heteronormativity, as long as it can be read culturally as heterocoital and homonormative. As long as Nic and Jules perform their parental roles according to gendered scripts, as long as they are a good enough imitation of the heterocoital family and the children know both biological genitors, as long as this homonormative ART-produced family successfully reproduces heterosexuality, the "kids are alright."

Private Life, a 2018 film by Tamara Jenkins, takes more risks in portraying reproductive mayhem caused by ARTs. It dwells in the messiness of gamete donation, surrogacy, and IVF's translation into heterocoital kinship configurations by showing characters who deal with probabilities and aftermath of donor conception that lead to familial chaos and insecure belonging. *Private Life* presents an interesting case because it compares adoption and ARTs and stages a debate about what is more "natural." At the center of this film's plot are Rachel (Kathryn Hahn) and Richard (Paul Giamatti), a married couple in their forties. Rachel, a playwright and novelist, and Richard, a former theater director, have built their lives and careers in the creative milieu of New York City. They are relatively successful as middle-class (they live in a rent-controlled apartment in the low-cost part of the East Village) and by bohemian standards (Richard is running an artisan pickle company while his theatrical career is on hiatus, and Rachel is about to publish a novel). They have been trying and failing to have a child for several years, including many cycles of IUI (intrauterine insemination), one failed attempt at domestic adoption, and a round of IVF "while waiting" for yet another adoption match. As the couple put it themselves, they are "trying to cover all the bases" because they are "not getting any younger." The film is an example of the "pursuit of fertility" plot, made grotesque by an absence of an explanation or reflection on why the couple wants a child. The film's laser focus on the couple's process of *getting* a child through seeking assisted reproductive technologies and adoption eclipses the usual thrust of the family drama toward portraying reproduction experiences as a matter of affective bonds developing between parents, children, and extended family. The focus on pursuit of fertility spotlights "the unnatural" in the couple's reproductive process and tests the limits of the audience's non-heterocoital reproduction acceptance.

The film begins with a scene that challenges the viewer's understanding of "natural" reproduction. Before anything appears on screen, we hear Richard saying, "Scoot over," and Rachel responding, "All right," in breathy, hushed voices. There are sighs and rustles, and the first image of Rachel's body suggests lovemaking: she is shot waist down, facing front, wearing skimpy bikini panties, her belly and legs exposed; Richard is climbing on the bed behind her, his hand on her hip, rolling her panties down. Yet it becomes clear within seconds that Richard is actually administering a painful fertility treatment shot. Rachel's unduly exposed flesh is no longer suggestive of sex; her belly now invokes images of pregnant women. The conversation between Richard and Rachel, who is complaining that the shot was too painful, is cut short by Richard, who says, "I'm not a doctor, remember?" While the image of Rachel's belly suggests the naturalness of pregnancy and human reproduction, Richard's words ending the scene ("I am not a doctor") emphasize the perceived *un*naturalness of what they are doing. By saying that he is not a doctor, Richard not only reminds Rachel that he is her partner and lover but also rejects the obvious intrusion of reproductive technology into the natural process of conception.

The film conveys the cultural "shame of being a fertility loser" (Clarke) by evoking sadness and embarrassment for the couple in the viewer. Both Richard and Rachel have their challenges: due to her age, Rachel is producing fewer viable eggs, while Richard has only one testicle and a sperm duct blockage. For Richard, the failure to procreate is a failure at traditional masculinity, which is further broken down into smaller-scale humiliations like his failure to achieve an erection while watching porn in the hospital specimen-retrieval room or to produce semen that has sperm in it. His embarrassment is accentuated by the tragicomic representations of his powerlessness and helplessness. For instance, he is struggling to turn off the porn video with a remote, which stops working at the worst possible time, and he has to shuffle over to the TV with his pants around his ankles and the paper seat-liner stuck to his rear end. The culmination of his "failures" is the scene of a fertilized egg transfer into Rachel's womb. The moment of possible conception does not include Richard. Rachel is in the procedure room with her fertility doctor, who likes to play prog rock during embryo implantation ("Say You Love Me" by John Lodge). Before he begins, the doctor smiles at her suggestively and says, "Let's get pregnant," in a tone that sounds almost seductive. This scene with the doctor, who sounds like her lover and the father of the child, is a reversal of the opening scene, in which Richard rejects the doctor's role. Such scene coupling seems to imply that the reproductive "failure" here is the absence of the coitus or conception link that would bring Rachel and Richard's genetic material together *naturally,* that is, in the fertility winners' way, which involves sexual penetration as a condition of conception. While such moments register as tragicomic, many critics observed that even the moments of comic relief in the film are marked with "sadness that is finally too thick to be cut by flashes of wit" (Edelstein). The "underlying feeling" of the film prompts the audience to react with pity or sympathy for Rachel and Richard, who are defeated by "how Nature works in an age when couples . . . wait so long to have kids" (Gleiberman). But Rachel and Richard's private "heartbreak" can also be seen as a proper punishment for not complying with nature and as a consequence of their individual failure to make the right reproductive choices at the right time (Gleiberman). In either case, the audience's emotional reaction serves to universalize the value of heterocoital reproduction and to associate adoption and ARTs with suffering and weirdness.

The lack of fertility invokes profound sadness, but so does the final choice the couple is left with—adoption. In *Private Life* adoption is associated with adoptive parents' potential emotional heartbreak as a result of the birth mother's decision to keep the child intended for adoption. But this archetypal fear takes a peculiar twist in this film. During their first attempt at adoption, the birth mother, with whom Rachel and Richard had been in contact for several months and whom they were supposed to meet at a diner in Arkansas around Christmas time, did not show up for the meeting. From an explanation they give to their new social worker, who visits them for an informal home study, it seems that Rachel and Richard attempted an individual adoption with no support from an adoption agency or a private attorney—the least common type. They did sign up with an adoption agency, but after two months of waiting for a match, they followed the advice of their former social worker to advertise themselves online as prospective parents. The birth mother called them, Skyped with them, told them the news about the baby's development, sent sonograms (no name or date on them), but broke off all contact after she had not shown for the planned meeting. Richard acknowledges to the social worker that they had been "warned against this stuff, but it's not like she asked . . . for money or anything," to which the social worker replies, "it's much easier when it involves money; at least that makes some kind of sense, but the emotional scams are just really, really tough." Adoption emotional scamming is indeed a phenomenon discussed in the adoption community, but the narrative choice of representing adoption through a relatively uncommon situation and the degree of cluelessness on Rachel and Richard's behalf about what the adoption process involves and proper ways of safeguarding it seems strange. It makes one wonder what purpose adoption serves in the narrative that focuses primarily on attempts to conceive a genetically continuous child.

As a plot device, adoption justifies Rachel and Richard's fixation on producing a genetically continuous child through its presentation as a better way to make a family. By becoming a "third-best choice" and serving as a foil to ARTs, adoption naturalizes IVF as enabling of heterocoital reproduction—IVF appears as a case of nature being "helped," not changed, by technology. Given the couple's history with adoption, IVF also appears to be a remedy for a potential birth-parent intrusion into the adoptive family structure. The final shot of the film solidifies this role of adoption. We see Rachel and Richard sitting side by side at an Applebee's, waiting for another birth mother. They have given up on biogenetic reproduction. As we watch, the scene that sets up expectations for a meeting with the birth mother gradually fades into the film's ending. Film credits are rolling over Rachel and Richard sitting at the table as the camera is slowly zooming out, and the viewers feel the uncertainty about the likelihood of this meeting happening. The viewers wonder if Rachel and Richard are in for yet another heartbreak. Even if it is possible to imagine that the birth mother is going to show up, the sadness permeating the scene is suggestive of seeing adoption as the "last resort." Such comparison of adoption and ARTs speaks to the idea of heterocoital reproduction primacy by revealing the preference for nontraditional reproduction that imitates the "real" one more seamlessly.

Yet, while it may seem that IVF assures a more seamless "passing" for a non-heterocoital family (after all, the genetic material may still come from the man and the woman who will be the parents of the child conceived this way), Franklin has observed in her interviews with IVF participants that "even people who succeed in the effort to achieve a take-home baby are often left disoriented and changed by their experience of undergoing IVF" (7). In the ways her interviewees are talking about IVF, Franklin notices a certain "ambivalence" that she attributes to "the difference between the norms that IVF belongs to, and the extent to which it also challenges or contradicts these very same conventions"—an effect that is not lost on those affected by the procedure, even though they may be struggling to name its source (7). In *Private Life,* this ambivalence is seen in the conflicting feelings experienced by the characters around different ways to have a child.

Rachel herself, as she is signing forms before her egg retrieval, says, "No, this is not normal, this is the opposite of normal." She is sitting in a hallway together with other couples—all men fully dressed, all women wearing the same hospital gowns and blue hairnets—a setting that foreshadows a later reference to *The Handmaid's Tale* (2017 series). The moment is ripe for an examination of IVF as a uniquely situated procedure, but Rachel continues with a rant about procreation by *any* means as unethical and names climate change, overpopulation, and so forth as reasons not to have children. The suggestive moment is reduced to a cliché and thus remains unexplored. The tug-of-war between seeing ARTs as a natural extension of heterocoital procreation as opposed to a freaky phenomenon with unknown consequences bubbles to the surface at other pivotal scenes in the film. The fertility doctor's suggestion to try egg donation as a procedure that has higher rates of success at Rachel's age is first met by her vehement rejection. The doctor's explanation describes the procedure as "a big leap" that has a significant "con"—"the loss of a genetic link for Rachel." To compensate for this perceived disadvantage, the doctor is trying to name a few "pros" that can help Rachel think of the potential baby as hers: she carries, controls the prenatal environment, gives birth, and breastfeeds, and Richard's genetic link is preserved. Yet Rachel sees "no way in hell [she's] doing that" and reminds Richard "that [they] decided as a couple that [they] would definitely draw the line at science fiction." More specifically, she objects to "putting somebody's body parts into [her] uterus." But the science fiction aspect Rachel perceives in ARTs seems to be also connected to the number of people (even if it is just their genetic material) involved in the process. IVF seems acceptable to her so long as it imitates biology of heterocoital reproduction and corresponds to the structure of a family that presumes two heterosexual genitors for a child. Rachel's quip "Why don't you [Richard] just go and screw a younger woman then?"—shows that in Rachel's thinking, conception and reproduction are firmly tied to coitus, even though she knows that the sex act is out of the picture in egg donation. Ultimately, Rachel reveals that she is upset because Richard will "have [his] genetic contribution" and she will "just be . . . left out." Her fear comes from a modernized version of "blood is thicker than water," an unexamined maxim very familiar to those involved in adoption, a cliché that presumes that an affective bond is an inevitable result of a biological-genetic connection.

Given that, Richard's response to Rachel's rejection of "science fiction" is interesting. He says, "We are already signed up for adoption. What is the big deal?" Adoption can hardly be characterized as science fiction, but together with Rachel's concern about letting other people's genetic material into her and Richard's child, the exchange may mean that the real issue here may be not the novelty of a procedure but the expanding nomenclature of family members having a direct genetic connection to the child. By splitting biological parenting from social, adoption challenges but still maintains the binary family structure: the child is transferred from its heterocoital origin into adoptive social parenting. In open adoption, the biological parent might be part of social parenting, but there is not much confusion about the child's heterocoital origin. A birth parent might be a threat to the integrity of adoptive family, but they are not a threat to the heterocoital order. In contrast, introducing biological material of a "stranger" into Rachel's body blurs the binary structure of heterocoital reproduction and, in turn, confuses the logic of kinship. Such a threat to the heterocoital order is experienced by Rachel as a threat to her parental ownership of the child. As she is trying to come to terms with egg donation, Rachel imagines that "it would be different if [she] had a younger sister or, like, a younger cousin, even, like, a family friend"—all these options seem more acceptable to her than accepting egg donation from a stranger. She explains her need for such "real connection" as the reason for her objection to "preying on the bodies of random young women," but the way she feels jealous when Richard talks about potential egg donors as attractive young women, and the decision of the couple to turn to IVF after a failed adoption attempt, may suggest that an explanation for Rachel's struggles over egg donation may be a bit more complex.

The part of the film in which Sadie, Rachel, and Richard's stepniece comes onto the stage as a prospective egg donor, troubles the neat "equivalency" of IVF and heterocoital reproduction that adoption (as a foil) helps to create. The concern about expanding the biological family structure beyond heterocoital in the process of using a donor egg is evident when Rachel is taken aback by Sadie's casual mentioning of "our baby." Rachel may read this phrasing as a presumption on Sadie's part that her genetic connection to the fetus gives her the right to the child or that at least there might be the need in the future to figure out how to manage this connection between Sadie and the child. Even when Rachel and Richard first approach Sadie "about her eggs," they trip over pronouns while explaining what will be put where:

> RACHEL: You would just go through, pretty much through what I just went through with IVF, minus the transfer.
> SADIE: What's the transfer?
> RICHARD: That's when they put the fertilized eggs back into your uterus.
> RACHEL: *My* uterus, in this case.
> RICHARD: Right, yes, yes, yes. It wouldn't be yours, because it would be Rachel's.

They may be talking about the uterus, but the conversation is also suggestive of questions around the ownership of the baby, which may be perceived as uncertain given the mixing of all parties' biological parts. In response to Richard's explanation that Sadie will have to do a psychiatric evaluation as a condition for being admitted into the egg donor program, Sadie jokes that it is done "so I don't go all Mary Beth Whitehead on you." She catches herself and dismisses as "creepy" the reference to a surrogate who refused to give the baby to the couple she was carrying the baby for. The joke is laughed off, but when Sadie, a budding writer, reveals to Rachel later that she is thinking of Rachel and Richard as her "art parents" and that it is going to get "more intense" because a part of her is going to be mixed with a part of him and growing inside Rachel, the prolonged shot of Rachel's face shows that she is bewildered and troubled.

She is not the only one trying to come to terms with the looming family structure (if the process works). Sadie's announcement about giving "the gift of life" to her aunt and uncle at her parents' Thanksgiving dinner is met with an awkward silence. Nobody is sure how to react to the news of a prospective "member of the family" created through such process. Even a sobriety speech by an alcoholic relative—who now seems like a more palatable black sheep in the family—cannot eclipse Sadie's news. Sadie's mother, Cynthia (Molly Shannon), exasperated, asks her daughter to consider what is going to happen after the baby is born, and Sadie replies that she could be Aunt Sadie or Cousin Sadie. But this answer does not satisfy her mother. Talking to her husband, Charlie (John Carroll Lynch), Cynthia complains that Sadie is "throwing around her genetic material like it's popcorn. Auctioning off family property like it's no big deal." Charlie answers that with "They are family. Richard and Rachel are family." This exchange is puzzling, and it is hard to understand what Charlie means. We see that he wants to protect Rachel and Richard's membership in the extended family in the absence of a direct biological connection (Richard is his stepbrother). But the very fact that Richard is not his "real" brother (read: genetically connected) makes using Sadie's eggs possible. Charlie slaps the placeholder concept of "family" on the messy kinship arrangement and the material circumstances of it as if there exists a tacit agreement on what "family" means and how this meaning explains this particular situation. Cynthia's remark brings up a whole host of questions about ownership of genetic material and its link to child ownership, but Charlie's answer cuts off this line of conversation by placing this instance of shared genetic material outside of the realm of material exchange. The proverbial can of worms full of intriguing questions about the consequences of ARTs is closed as soon as it is opened, though. And in the end, the film neutralizes these unfolding contradictions by denying the possibility of any unconventional family arrangement. The egg donation process is portrayed as a failed reproductive attempt. Rachel and Richard return to adoption, a more familiar cultural script in which the heterosexual genitors of a child are implied even if not known.

Even though it presents the messiness of kinship, *Private Life* is not going as far as suggesting ways of dealing with it. Instead, it reestablishes the inevitability of the link between shared genetics and attachment that sustains the cultural script of heterocoital family primacy. Rachel and Richard's inability to have a genetically continuous family is represented as a profound loss of genetic and affective attachment that their own relationship, adoption, or their relationship with Sadie (who seems like a daughter to them) cannot compensate for. As it attempts to "naturalize" assisted reproduction, the film showcases the discursive aspect of biology, which can now be reimagined as a process rather than a fact. Through failing reinscriptions of heterocoital kinship terms onto IVF and gamete donation, it exposes the narrative excess of non-heterocoital forms of reproduction that cannot be neatly packaged in traditional family terms and points to the need for revisions of cultural ideas we can use to think through new forms of reproduction and kinship.

All four films discussed in this chapter, some directly, and some via intricate reasoning footwork, reaffirm heterocoital kinship even as they reveal incongruities created where heterocoital frameworks clash against adoption and ARTs experience. They demonstrate that "whether by adoption or by technological innovation . . . artificially achieved families certainly rewrite the originary place of the blood tie for those growing up outside of their biological bloodline. However, even within these radical ways of achieving family, the kinship origin remains a foundational source of knowledge and truth" (Sales 8). The move toward universalization of reproductive experience by imagining all reproduction as heterocoital is sustained by the ethos of the melodrama genre. Gledhill and Williams observe that "to touch its audiences' lives, melodrama has to command recognition, whether of human feeling, social experience, or moral dilemma" (10). They explain that such recognition may extend not only to culturally common phenomena but also to "classes of people, of social conditions, or of areas of life hitherto unrepresented," and that melodrama achieves this by constantly challenging "codes of verisimilitude and thus changing the way reality is perceived and understood" (10). Melodrama brings into the cultural imaginary new ways of being, but their legibility depends on their resonance with what is already recognized. In nontraditional kinship narrative, such recognition of the previously unknown is achieved through attachment of a recognizable structure of feeling to the new form of reality. For the majority of the viewers, empathy for someone defined by reproductive difference is contingent on reading it as akin to heterocoital identity and life trajectory, since we understand the new in terms of the already known, which means that we understand one thing in terms of another, in other words, metaphorically.[12] By soliciting recognition of non-heterocoital family formations through the use of familiar heterocoital tropes, adoption, and ARTs, melodramas produce reproductive difference at

12. As in Lakoff and Johnson; also see Strathern on the pitfalls of understanding one thing in terms of another.

the moment of creating pathways for its cultural acceptance. In this way, even as it acquaints the viewers with nontraditional reproduction and kinship, it pulls the viewers into affective work that reproduces heterocoital structures of feeling as the culturally desirable moral order and reinscribes them onto the new reproductive contexts.

CHAPTER 2

Adoption and ARTs in Horror Film

The Hidden Spring of Heterocoital Origin

Abject and abjection are my safeguards. The primers of my culture.

—Kristeva, *Powers of Horror* (2)

While nontraditional reproduction drama shows that the deep-seated cultural need to stabilize the origin of a child as heterocoital is interdependent with the cultural insistence on monomaternalism and cultural preference for the heterocoital family, the horror genre makes the reasons for such stabilizing visible. It reveals the fears and anxieties Western cultures keep churning in response to non-heterocoital kinship and reproduction. To assuage these anxieties, the emotional landscapes of adoption and ARTs horror films foster the viewers' affective stances that support cultural insistence on heterocoital family as a site of secure futurity. In general, the horror genre "challenge[s] our commonplace assumptions about safety and security" and reminds us of the value of the social order by "making us aware of the ways in which we have constructed a safe worldview in order to function" (Fahy 5). The thrill and pleasure of horror is in the experience of discovering and defeating a monster and a return to the "safety net of predictability" in what is accepted as the real world (Fahy 12). The experience of viewing films about evil adoptees or technohorrors of assisted reproduction acclimates the viewers to culturally acceptable stances on breaches of kinship normalcy. Such viewing creates experiences of fear and disgust with a being or a way of life that "represent[s] . . . unmapped areas bordering the familiar configurations of the social world" (Prince 122), for example, with the adoptee challenging the ethos of the heterocoital nuclear family with their reproductive difference. Together with aversion to breaches of normalcy, the pleasures of horror cinema orient the viewer toward socially desirable structures of feeling. The emotions of anxiety, disgust, and fear endured by the viewer of a horror film are not an end in themselves but "part of the price to be paid" for the pleasure of discovering and defeating the monster (Carroll 184). A significant component of this pleasure, according to Noel Carroll is "the process of . . . ratiocination" that can begin once the monster is recognized (184). Carroll points out that the loathsomeness of monsters comes from their "being interstitial" and thus "'unknown'" (185), and the pleasure of their discovery may come from understanding "the ways they violate our classificatory scheme" (185).[1]

For example, the adoptee's simultaneous attachment to different genealogies challenges our conceptual schema of kinship and reproduction in which nature and nurture coincide and reliably reproduce culturally safe, homogenous genealogical lineages. The thrill of adoption horror thus often comes from the adoptees "passing" as regular human children that can be expected to share our culture, and the viewers' pleasure comes from the explanation of the adoptee's abjection via a discovery of the adoptees' secret origins that connect them to something culturally abnormal or evil. An ARTs horror film may tantalize with the uncertainty of the reproductive process, which can be portrayed as resulting in reproduction of monsters or as being controlled by monsters. An evil doctor or scientist who is pursuing their own goals and using an unsuspecting mother-to-be as a guinea pig, or a child who blurs the boundaries between animals and humans or humans and technology, are among the common tropes in ARTs horror. The library of adoption horror films is larger than that of those featuring assisted reproduction, probably because ARTs have been largely relegated to the sci-fi genre, which typically hosts less "real" subject matter. However, the recent interest in what an article in *The Economist* calls "reproductive techno-horror" points to the transition of ARTs into the category of more "real" threats that are being treated now within a genre that is more interested in neutralizing them and is more culturally conservative than sci-fi.[2] This chapter lingers on adoption horror films to unpack the challenges of the non-heterocoital origin of a child, and especially of a lack of knowledge about it, to a social order built around

1. Prince, too, suggests not just paying attention to the ways the horror genre produces affective responses of fear on an individual psychological level but also to how these responses depend on perceived breakdowns of the social and natural orders. In *The Horror Film* chapter "Dread, Taboo, and the Thing," Prince says that various interpretations of the meaning of the genre rely on the same "connecting logic": their imagery and effects are understood as "manifestation[s] of psychic processes . . . projections or displacements of fears or as signifiers of a cultural state of mind" (118). Such explanation directly connects affect and culture.

2. See "Reproductive Techno-Horror Is a Burgeoning Genre on Screen."

heterocoital reproduction. Then it examines ART horror films, which more vividly demonstrate the patriarchy's investment in heterocoital reproduction, in its successful imitations, and, when this fails, in total control over the process of assisted reproduction.

•

Portrayals of the adoptee's unknown origins in adoption horror film help us understand what exactly about nontraditional kinship may be perceived as threatening by cultures structured around heterocoital reproduction and kinship. While in melodrama the lack of or uncertainty about heterocoital origin is portrayed as a source of private, individual melancholia, adoption horror film focuses on portraying the threat presented by the origins of the adoptee to the wider community and nation. Unlike melodrama that engages with interior lives of non-heterocoital family members, adoption horror takes a public turn and taps into the emotions of fear and disgust, foundational to the genre,[3] in order to set up a private conflict between the evil adoptee and the victimized adoptive family as a confrontation with a social ripple effect. The impact of the adoptees' unknown or concealed origins spills into the community, and it is not uncommon to see agents of the social order (nuns, priests, social workers, police officers, journalists) die at the hands of the "evil adoptee." The adoptive family has to take a side in this conflict and resolve it by killing or banishing the adoptee. If the adoptive family still believes that the adoptee can be integrated into the social fabric and insists on loving the "monster," the ending may remain ambiguous, and the final sequence may suggest a lingering threat.

Adoption horror responds to questions about adoption that are implied, even if not voiced, in Western cultural ideas about non-heterocoital kinship. It reorients one of the main ones—"Can you love this child as your own?"—toward "Can this child love you like your own?" In other words, the horror genre engages with the cultural anxiety about the loyalty of the adopted person to their family, community, and nation, an anxiety rooted in understanding cultural transmission as tethered to heterocoital reproduction. Paradoxically, though, the horror genre is not that concerned with the psychic processes of adoptees. The adoptee point of view is practically absent in the horror genre, and the recovery of origins is typically done not by the adoptees themselves but by the adoptive parents, who want to understand "what is wrong" with their child. The knowledge of origins thus does not involve a

3. See the discussion of these two emotions' roles in the horror aesthetic in Carroll.

reunion with the biological family. In adoption horror, the birth parents tend to remain erased and reduced to biogenetic-heterocoital origin knowledge that explains the adoptee's wickedness. The search for origins unfolds not as a discovery of an adoptee's past or its acknowledgment for the sake of personal and family healing, as in melodrama, but as what Noel Carroll calls a "complex discovery plot"—a typical horror genre narrative structure that involves a discovery of a monster, with its subsequent "confirmation and confrontation" (99). The answer to the question "Can the adopted child love the adoptive family and community as their own?" is practically always a "no."

Within such plots, the adoptee is not an innocent possessed child whose depravity is the work of evil spirits or demons that can be exorcised. The origins of the evil adoptee are already marked by a loss of innocence as, for example, in *The Bad Seed,* a 1956 film based on a National Book Award–nominated novel by William March. *The Bad Seed* is often recognized as the first example of the cinematic adoption horror genre. In the film, the evil skips a generation and comes out as psychopathic tendencies transferred through an adoptee, Christine Penmark (Nancy Kelly), to her biological daughter, Rhoda (Patty McCormack). Rhoda, an angelic nine-year-old brought up in a loving family, is capable of murder without remorse. The source of her pathology is her genetic connection to her grandmother, Christine's biological mother, who was a psychopathic killer. Cynthia Callahan points out the genetic determinism of this narrative, which constructs "the concept of the 'bad seed,' a child whose negative hereditary traits will unleash chaos on an unsuspecting family" (1). The concept of the unknown genetic threat that "lingers around adoption" (Callahan 1) is at the core of adoption horror that focuses on "evil-by-nature" adoptees. This intractable encoding of evil into the child may also be represented as an adoptee's hidden disability, as in Jaume Collet-Serra's *Orphan* (2009), or as lingering consequences of early childhood trauma that resists rehabilitation, as in *Luce* (2019).[4] In cases of trauma-induced wickedness, "origins" may be understood as a pre-adoption past marked by neglect and a failure of the birth family to preserve the innocence of the child.

The conflicts of adoption horror film originate in the assumption of the adoptee's untrustworthiness, which is a consequence of their incapacity for the affect that holds families and communities together. The contrast between the child's innocent appearance and their violent affect and behavior underscores

4. *Luce* is not a horror film in the classical meaning of the genre; it does not contain supernatural elements or an openly murderous adoptee. It is a psychological thriller, but I find it worth including in this discussion because it follows the logic of the horror film yet offers a more subtle portrayal of the sources of psychological horror associated with the figure of the adoptee in the horror genre.

the threat posed by the adoptees' reproductive difference, which cannot be immediately detected and then managed by the adoptive family. By showing communities damaged by the adoptive family's inability to control the adoptee's hidden lack of acceptable affect, the horror genre underscores the social responsibility of the adoptive parents for the correct socialization of the child into forms of affect and behavior that make the adoptee a loyal conduit of the adoptive culture. In other words, adoption horror conflicts suggest that, in the absence of heterocoital connection to the adoptive community, an adoptee may not become a reliable conduit of its culture and a solid block in the symbolic order. The adoptee's reproductive difference remains a threat that nurture fails to control.

The adoptee terrorizing the adoptive family and community is a variation on the "evil child" genre—a relatively recent phenomenon in literature and film. In her study of children in the horror genre, Sabine Bussing observes that, as a literary character, the child emerged as a subject in Romantic poetry at the end of the eighteenth century, "when poets began to regard not only the adult mind, but also the feelings" that were associated with free emotional expression in children (xiii). She and several other scholars[5] observe that since the beginning of this emotional turn, "childhood came to be treasured as a metaphor for the ideal human condition" and the child gained a more prominent role in literature (xiii). By the twentieth century, "the child has become absolutely indispensable" to the horror genre, transforming into "a frequent aggressor, killer, and a veritable monster" (Bussing xiv), and the end of the twentieth and beginning of the twenty-first centuries saw a boom of evil child text production (Renner 2013). The child, characterized by innocence but also by drives unconstrained by reason, has become a productive horror genre character suitable for the exploration of the disciplining of emotions, affect, and irrationality as a matter of being human.

As a being unconstrained by reason, the child is often understood as a transitional figure between human and animal, a site of socialization and domestication. When defined as "not animal," the child is imagined as affectively unstable, not in control of impulses and drives that need to be disciplined in order for the child to engage in social exchanges in the ways acceptable by culture. The horror genre taps into the cultural idea that a child is not completely human but "a border identity" and a "limit case" of "affiliation to the human" (Fuss 5).[6] Diana Fuss explains that a child's humanity is

5. For example, Prince.

6. See also a cluster of essays on children by Cora Kaplan, James Kincaid, and Drucilla Cornell in the collection edited by Diana Fuss, *Human, All Too Human*.

an elastic concept constructed by "political ideology, cultural mythology, legal doctrine, and social policy" and is thus dependent upon the contemporaneous cultural meanings of humanity (5). The exploration of evil and monstrous child representations, then, is an opportunity to observe what idea of humanity is constructed at a specific historical moment and how it is determined by social forces. In his study of the horror genre, Stephen Prince looks at the child in this light as he aims to expand Robin Wood's psychoanalytical reading of the horror genre as the return of the repressed and as "mirroring the projection of [individual] psychological demons" (129). By shifting the focus from understanding horror genre conflicts as individual and private, Prince draws attention to the social function of horror, which "addresses the persistent question of what must be done to remain human" within the mutually constitutive relationship between an individual and the social world (129). Prince thus believes that banishment of the monster—a typical resolution to a horror plot—is not only an exorcism of personal demons but a process that serves to reinforce "the validity and arrangement of the established social categories" (129). Prince's emphasis on studying the social implications of the genre suggests engagement of the psychic processes by social structures. In this case, cinematic horror can be understood as a breakdown of cultural scripts by someone—a child—who cannot or will not participate in the affective order that ensures the continuity of the symbolic, social order.

A child can only achieve a fully human, autonomous status after socialization is complete, and the child's capacity for socially acceptable affect is one of the conditions of inclusion into the world of adults. Until then, the child remains a responsibility of their parents, construed as someone in need of protection and control, and the perpetual infantilization of the adoptee may point to the cultural uncertainty about the possibility to fully integrate or discipline a person with reproductive difference. Such concerns are central to horror films that explore affective aberrations or manifestations of undisciplined affect in children. The taxonomies of evil children, developed by Karen J. Renner and Andrew Scahill, show that cultural concerns around the humanity of a child imagine the child's affect as aberrant if it is sub- or non-human (animalistic, demon-like) or more-than-human (wise beyond one's years and able to understand and manipulate adults without revealing its own motives). The absence of affective responses is also imagined as an aberration. Bussing, for example, observes "a strangely flat impression" of the evil child who lacks "individual traits and qualities" in comparison to the figure of the child in other genres (xiv), and Scahill reserves a category—the watcher—for a child whose innocence may also be read as emptiness waiting to be "filled up with noninnocent qualities" (16). The concern with the child's capacity for the right kind of affect is persistent in the horror narratives that use the figure of the child to work out what makes us socially functioning humans.

This concern with the children's affective capacity as a matter of being human is persistently coupled with the concern about their ability to assure uninterrupted futurity. By revealing the monstrous inhumanity of the child, who becomes "a vessel for all the fears that concern the existence of Man" (Bussing xv), the horror film invites the viewer to recognize and feel the importance of genealogical and cultural continuity that a *child-becoming-human* provides to the world that needs to be held together. The birth of a child is a promise of futurity, a countermove to physical and cultural entropy, so a glitch in the process of a *child-becoming-future*—such as an unknown or "wrong" origin coupled with a failure to feel and act in socially acceptable ways—threatens to upend the symbolic order that a *child-becoming-adult* is supposed to maintain. Adoption horror shows that desirable futurity depends on the child being reliably, predictably human in the sense of having their known heterocoital origin coupled with the capacity for the right kind of affect that serves to maintain and perpetuate social structures and structures of feeling based on heterocoital kinship, even if they are enacted by its as-if heterocoital forms. Such values determine what child can be a part of the family and what family can have a child. Andrew Scahill's analysis, for example, looks at children in the horror genre as queer figures that channel "familial dissociation: some children adopted and returned to the family, some other children—'Othered' children—remaining forever foreign, and still others troubling the boundaries and coherence of kinship itself" (84). By including films like *Orphan, Silent Hill* (2006), or *The Ring* (2002) in the category of films featuring "unwanted" children, Scahill comes close to the discussion of adoption in the horror genre (85–86). His analysis reads adoption as a symbolic gesture within horror plots that feature the return of a victimized child as a ghost. Such a child tortures families until the child's trauma is discovered and recognized and the ghost is "adopted" by the adults that "recupera[te]" the child's past and innocence by "restor[ing]" the child "into the patriarchal order" (89). Scahill also looks at the category of "unadoptable" children within horror plots, who "have no place within the discursive formation of childhood" and are "unable to be restored to the symbolic order" (91). He connects such figures of children to culture's resistance to queering of kinship, including gay adoption in the literal sense as well as in the sense of the chosen family (non-heterocoital kinship), and observes that recuperated ghost children, who "work to reassert the ascendancy of the present over the past," suggest the enduring power of the family to restore the child to goodness (89). In other words, the symbolic adoption of the ghost child conserves and reasserts the cultural value of the heterocoital family: "the family may be the problem (generations ago), but the family is also the solution (today, forever forward)" (89).

The figure of the ghost child, whose spirit leaves after the story of their past trauma is discovered by the haunted, seems to overlap with adoption drama's theme of healing through origin recovery. But this horror scenario erases rather than engages with adoption. The adoptive parents stop being parents after the ghost child is satisfied with the recognition of their past, and the safety of the community is restored only after the disappearance of the child. Scahill acknowledges that such plots do not dwell on something "so messy and complicated as true accommodation within family" (89), since, after the ghost child's "releas[e] from the miasma of unknowingness" and symbolic adoption by the "surroga[te]" parents, she "conveniently evaporate[s]" (89). A ghost child scenario that comes closer to engaging adoption might be the one in which the ghost with recovered origin trauma remains attached and follows the surrogate adoptive family, as in the franchises of *The Grudge* and *The Ring*. In these cases, the children's known origins never fully restore them to innocence, and they continue to haunt and spread the curse to increasing numbers of people. They often possess or eliminate biological children of the surrogate adoptive "parents," since they are blindly driven by the need for love and nurture and do not want to share these resources with anyone else. Yet, they are never satisfied with the acknowledgment or love they receive, and they remain forever hungry ghosts, truly unrecoverable children who do not respond to attempts to help them. They cannot love appropriately, and their unchecked affect inevitably destroys the adoptive family, so they have to move on to the next one. The presence of such an adoptee in the adoptive family thus takes the form of an uncontainable threat not only to the family but also to the larger community. In such narratives, the collective futurity is compromised by the adoptee's origin, which destroys or permanently others the adoptive family and community.

A similar plot logic is traceable in the narratives where the evil adoptee is embodied and adoption is taken literally rather than symbolically. Such cases may still feature the attribution of the adoptee's wickedness to early trauma (more about this later), but narratives where adoption is literal also show concern over the impact of the origins on the child's capacity for the right kind of affect. This concern is often manifested by grounding the wickedness of the adoptee in the adoptee's body and its reproductive history. Damien in *The Omen* is a son of the devil and a jackal mother. Rhoda in *The Bad Seed* is a granddaughter of a serial killer. Even the adoptee whose incapacity for the right affect is caused by trauma often cannot be rehabilitated because there is a reproductive problem at the level of the body. Alessa's body in *Silent Hill* is split by rape into her innocent and evil manifestations, which function as two different girls, and their eventual reunification does not restore the adoptive family but separates its timelines and futurities. Esther's body in *Orphan* is marked by hereditary dwarfism—a condition that makes her look like a permanent child. While in itself this disability is not necessarily connected to affective disorders, the film portrays it as a possible cause of Esther's wickedness. She uses her condition to her advantage, but she also suffers from it, as it forecloses the possibility of reproduction and frustrates her attempts at a desired heterocoitus with an adult male. In *Luce*, the adoptive father is wondering if all the problems brought onto their family by their adopted son could have been avoided if he and his wife had reproduced heterocoitally—if their child's body was biologically connected to their reproductive history. The embodied adoptee of the horror genre thus opens up avenues into exploring the role reproductive difference and affect have in determining one's humanity as a guarantee of continuous and possible social futurity. Adoption horror suggests that heterocoital origin determines the success of becoming human, both biologically and socially, and that a break in heterocoital genealogy undermines desirable futurity (i.e., successful reproduction of culture), represented by a naturally reproduced and correctly socialized child. Adoptees' failure to successfully imitate heterocoital reproduction understood as such typically leads to their expulsion from the family and community in films' endings that are meant to be "happy."

In horror films that imagine the origin of adoptees' wickedness as their evil nature—that is, as a heterocoital, genetic transfer of evil from the biological parents—the conflict is likely to be resolved by the adoptees' death at the hands of their adoptive or surrogate parents, or by an act of god or nature. This violence is meant to be experienced by the viewer as pleasurable since the death of the evil child is equated with restored safety via an erasure of the "faulty" genealogical line that reproduces evil and hides itself in adoption. Such ending is supposed to console the viewer with a reinstatement of the cultural belief in heterocoital kinship's ability to predict which bodies will reproduce which values. The plot, in which the adoptee's wickedness is attributed to early trauma as opposed to genetic flaws, may remain at the stage of a normalizing "ratiocination" (Carroll 184) of the adoptee's behavior. In this latter case, the adoptee usually remains a member of the adoptive family, even though their goodness is still in question. The viewers may feel a lingering anxiety at the end of such films due to the continuing uncertainty about the outcome of nontraditional reproduction or kinship. Such an ending, however, opens up space for cognitive distancing that facilitates a more complex response to the violation of acceptable cultural schemas by adoption. The viewer may be drawn into considering the complexities of an adoption situation, even if the film leans on its dangers.

The classic of adoption horror, *The Bad Seed,* belongs to the category of narratives that attribute adoptee's wickedness to their genetic origin. In such narratives, the evil is imagined as hereditary, intractable, and inevitable. Christine Ward Gailey writes that *Bad Seed* "ushered in a 'demon child' adoption formula" that eventually collapsed the scenario of "evil skipping a generation" and resulted in representations of adoptees as "the embodiment of evil" (74). Gailey places *The Bad Seed* (1956) with the "Red Scare" wave of 1950s films, "a memorable spate of 'enemy within' horror films" in which the enemy looked "like any(white)one, but deep within [was] inherently murderous" (73). She observes that the source of Rhoda's evil—the unknown origins of the adoptee—is a reflection of the tension between cultural preoccupation with "eugenics" combined with "the reality of sealed adoption records," which, together, bred the fear of "natural born killers" that can pass for normal children (73). The generation skip may be pointing as well to the connection of this plot to the racial passing narrative, in which the discovery of the white-presenting passer happens after the birth of their Black child. The heterocoital origin of the child becomes evidence of passing and the reason for the passer's banishment from the safety of white domesticity. By the logic of the passing narrative, both mother and daughter in *Bad Seed* are trespassers of the social order. The unsuspecting adoptee-passer, Christine Penmark, is punished as much as the actual psychopathic killer. When she learns about her origin, she strikes her womb, which, in her mind, is the cause of the horror unleashed by Rhoda on their community. Her own reproductive "success" as a "normal" child of a serial killer does not matter—in this scenario, she is a social passer and a passer of the evil gene, who will be punished with the destruction of the bloodline all the way back to the dead serial killer mother. The resolution Christine chooses—murder suicide—underscores the narrative's insistence on destroying the adoptee, a glitch in traceable genealogy that otherwise could have prevented Rhoda's birth. While not directly engaged with the theme of racial passing, *The Bad Seed* draws on the logic of the passing narrative, which may suggest that, at its core, the conflict of adoption horror is about a clash of two cultures warring to reproduce themselves through an adoptee's body. For this reason, the transnational adoptee[7] and adoptee-passer often become central characters of adoption horror that make conspicuous the

7. Or "transcultural," in John McLeod's (2015) terminology.

cultural importance of biological origin in American culture.[8] The adoption horror film also underscores that we cannot equate nurture with guaranteed transfer of culture; instead, we need to triangulate the process of reproduction (nature—nurture—culture) in order to understand cultural resistance to nontraditional kinship as a resistance to culture hybridization.

By separating nurture and nature sites in the reproduction process, adoption shows to what extent heterocoital kinship informs belonging—understood as the ability to live and transmit unhybridized culture—not only at the level of the adoptive family but also at the level of community and nation. For example, genealogy—alongside and often more so than visual difference or nonbiological kinship relations (such as marriage and adoption)—has played a major role in racialized social stratification of bodies in segregated America. Narratives that trouble the assumption of cultural continuity through heterocoital reproduction, for example, narratives of passing and adoption, bring into high relief the foundational characteristic of American culture—the clash between its preoccupations with descent and the ideal of self-invention.[9] Writing about the cultural paradoxes behind the American idea of adoption, Judith Modell explains how this clash manifests in the adoption context. She points out that the idea of adoption as a "contracted relationship" that assumes "the achievement of identity" and "the possibility of *making oneself*" has not been "comfortable in American culture" or law, which insist on the concept of the "as if begotten" adoptive family (182). Modell sees in this concept "a contradiction between core cultural values: respecting the 'nature' of a person and granting a person the freedom to construct an identity" (182), which is a double bind that adoptees and adoptive families have to contend with when accommodating the adoptee's pre-adoption past in their narratives of belonging. Adoption horror taps into these conflicting ideas when it presents adoption as a "cover-up" that precludes knowledge of the child's biological origin—a threat posed by the reproductive difference of the adoptee to the adoptive family and larger community.

The Omen franchise (1976–2006) is an example of thinking that imagines the threat of a genetically different and evil child reaching beyond the adoptive family and becoming a threat to national security and humanity at large. In the 1976 film, Damien (Harvey Stephens) is adopted by an American couple, Robert (Gregory Peck) and Katherine Thorn (Lee Remick) in Rome. Robert, an American diplomat, is approached by a chaplain at the hospital

8. Narratives that couple passing, which depends on concealed ancestry, and adoption, which often precludes the knowledge of descent, reveal the cultural significance of (un)known genealogy. See Fedosik 2009a.

9. See Singley on connections between adoption, self-invention, and Americanism.

where his wife has given birth and told that his son was stillborn. The chaplain suggests that Robert adopt another newborn, whose mother died at birth, and conceal it from Katherine. Robert is the only parent who knows about adoption, even though Katherine eventually begins to suspect that something is wrong with her son. After a few strange domestic events, several gruesome killings including of Katherine's second unborn child, and several warnings, Robert sets out to find information about Damien's origin. He goes back to Italy and eventually discovers that Damien is not biologically human; he is a son of a jackal mother and Satan himself. The recovered heterocoital origin explains his wickedness as a consequence of his inhuman nature; his passing as a human is a threat to the whole of humanity. Robert understands that he has to kill Damien and rid the world of the threat. Yet, Damien looks like a vulnerable human boy, and it makes his father hesitate. The hesitation has a terrible cost. In the end, Katherine is killed by Damien's nanny, Robert is shot by the police, Damien survives, and the film ends with him grinning at the camera at his parents' funeral. His hand is held by the President of the United States, which suggests a threat to the American nation. Such an ending extends the reach of Damien's origin to the national and global level and, as Gailey observes, contributes to "the image of international adoptees as sociopaths-in-waiting" (76). Gailey points to the pervasive use of the transnational adoptee as a threatening figure when she observes that "the theme of international adoptee as a sociopath continues in horror films to the present even as few movies outside this genre focus on dynamics of international adoption" (76). A consideration of *The Bad Seed* and *The Omen* as belonging to the same genre of adoption horror points to a continuity between the passing narrative, the 1950s Red Scare narratives about foreigners living undetected in our midst (Gailey 74), and the narratives of evil transnational adoptees. All of them are preoccupied with discovering otherness that is hiding in plain sight, an otherness that is threatening because it disrupts the synergy of biological, cultural, and national reproduction. As a "cover" for unknown, uncertain, wrongly identified, or concealed heterocoital origins, adoption puts the loyalty of the adopted person to their family, culture, nation, and even humanity in question. The reaction to this threat, which often manifests as an obsession with the adoptee's capacity for the right affect and loyalty to the adoptive family, is also understood as the capacity for loyalty to the adoptive community and nation at large. Horror films about transnational adoptees doubt this capacity and ask whether the adopted foreign child could be turned into a loyal citizen of the adoptive nation. Films discussed later in this chapter, *Orphan* and *Luce,* also explore what can go wrong in this process by representing transnational adoptions gone wrong or, in the case of *Luce,* as uncertain.

Several scholars have pointed out that one of the most important functions of the transnational adoptive family in American culture has been signification of a tolerable, middle-class diversity, sanctioned by the American immigration legislation.[10] As a lawful immigrant successfully assimilated into American culture, the adoptee has been setting an example of legal immigration into the US, and the adoptive family was called upon to demonstrate the power of a middle-class (mostly white) American family to socialize an immigrant child into a loyal citizen. The wayward transnational adoptee of the horror genre is the foil of the adoptee as a model immigrant. The adoption horror genre often draws on the cultural fear of assimilation gone wrong and engages with disrupted or problematic transnational adoption. It engages the cultural idea of adoptive parenting as a civic duty that keeps the community and nation safe by controlling and eliminating the potential threats presented by a disloyal adoptee. Both *Orphan* and *Luce* present central conflicts built around the adoptive family's inability to correctly socialize the adoptee and manage their undisciplined affect and questionable loyalty. While *Luce* offers a more nuanced negotiation of an adoptee's hybrid identity and belonging, *Orphan* approaches the subject with the bluntness of an adoption exploitation film.[11]

The source of horror in *Orphan* is the unknown origin of an Eastern European adoptee, Esther (Isabelle Fuhrman). The film is informed by representations of the Eastern European adoptee in larger American popular culture, which, at the time of its production, frequently invoked the image of the psychologically disturbed or otherwise disabled child. Even though the adoption community may have had a more nuanced understanding of the specific character of Eastern European adoptions, the coverage of such adoptions in the media often focused on adoption disruption and the qualities of the adoptees that might have made them unadoptable. Specifically, *Orphan* is an heir to the category of disrupted Eastern European adoption narratives that center on the child with a "hidden problem—the specter of the pretty, physically 'normal,' and apparently healthy child . . . who could not be saved by compassionate action" (Cartwright 202). In her article "Images of 'Waiting Children,'" Lisa Cartwright observed a trend in perceptions of Eastern European adoptions—mostly Romanian—which in "the 1990s began with transnational news stories and a transnational humanitarian movement dedicated to saving the global social orphan, the child at risk in states incapable of providing adequate

10. See Dorow; Nelson on the ideological meaning of adoption in the context of immigration.

11. Kim Park Nelson introduced this term at the 2010 Alliance for the Study of Adoption and Culture (ASAC) conference.

care and protection" and "ended with the rescue fantasy gone awry" when it became clear that a significant number of adopted children were developing behavioral, cognitive, and developmental problems, sometimes serious enough to endanger the well-being or even lives of their adoptive family members (201–2). The cultural sources of *Orphan*'s horror scenario can also be traced back to several sensationalized American cases of disrupted Eastern European adoptions, such as Artyom Savelyev's—the boy who was "sent back" to Russia by his American adoptive mother, who could not cope with his behavior (see Stewart).

The prominence of disrupted Eastern European adoption representations and their sensationalist character may be partially explained by the fact that monoracial Eastern European adoptions that have "worked"—by the standards of the adoptive culture, family, and community—rarely gained post-adoption visibility in popular American culture. At the turn of the twenty-first century, Eastern European adoptions became popular because they offered several advantages over domestic adoptions or transnational adoptions from other regions. In addition to the well-recognized advantage of the legally secured birthparent's absence in (legal) transnational placements, the ongoing popularity of Eastern European adoptions "might [have] be[en] explained . . . by the 'racial' preferences of [white] adoptive parents" (Khabibullina 174). Racial matching gave Eastern European adoptees and their white adoptive families more control over their adoptive status disclosure—a freedom unavailable to transracial families, who have to deal with "interracial surveillance" on a daily basis (Jacobson 2008, 146). Stories of disrupted adoption couple the advantages of this kind of "passing" with anxiety over the child's possible hidden disabilities that can disrupt the seamless integration of the adoptee and adoptive family in the adoptive culture and community. And while many visible physical disabilities have been perceived as acceptable, hidden disabilities and mental health issues that may undermine the development of the child's expected affect (as in Savelyev's case) have been grounds enough for adoption disruption.

Orphan comes to terms with such anxiety over the presence of the "unsalvageable" child in American culture, family, and community. It explores the cultural fear of hidden impairments that place the unsalvageable adoptee beyond the normalizing reach of the American family. Hidden disabilities dwelling in the body of the (supposedly) nine-year-old adoptee Esther are exposed as reasons for havoc she wreaks on the family of Kate and John Coleman (Vera Farmiga and Peter Sarsgaard), a white, middle-class couple with two biological children, their hearing-impaired daughter, Max, and their son, Daniel. The family adopt Esther from a Catholic orphanage in the US after

Kate gives birth to a stillborn baby. The Colemans are told that Esther was initially adopted from Russia by another American couple, but she has lived in St. Mariana's orphanage since her first adoptive family perished in a fire. Esther attracts the Colemans by emotional maturity, unusual for her age, and artistic gifts—she is a talented painter. After the initial adjustment period at her new home, Esther's psychopathic tendencies begin to emerge: she severely injures a girl who teases her in school, terrorizes Max (Aryana Engineer) and Daniel (Jimmy Bennett), and kills Sister Abigail (C. C. H. Pounder)—a nun from the orphanage who threatens to remove Esther from the Colemans' home and warns Kate that "trouble has a way of finding Esther." Esther is a talented enough manipulator to make the aftermath of her violent outbursts look like accidents, so while Kate is becoming progressively suspicious of her adopted daughter and is trying to find out about her past, John and the family therapist refuse to recognize signs of trouble; they find Kate, a former alcoholic, unstable and untrustworthy.

Esther's manipulations, aimed at securing the love and protection of her "Daddy," undermine Kate's role as the mother. In an especially cruel manipulation, in order to provoke Kate's anger and make her look violent and unhinged, Esther cuts down the roses that Kate planted in the greenhouse as a memorial to her stillborn baby, Jessica. At the end of the film, after many spine-chilling psychopathic escapades, Esther succeeds in putting Daniel and Kate in the hospital in order to arrange an intimate moment at home with her adoptive father. Wearing Kate's black lace dress and heavy makeup, Esther attempts to seduce John, who finally recognizes that "there is something wrong with Esther" and threatens to "re-consider her future" in his family in the morning. The threat triggers Esther's killing spree: she stabs John to death and nearly kills Max and Kate, who has rushed home from the hospital after getting a call from a doctor at the Saarne Institute, a mental hospital in Estonia. The doctor reveals that Leena (Esther's real name) is a violent and extremely dangerous patient of theirs, not an orphan from Russia. A more shocking revelation, though, is that Leena, in fact, is thirty-three years old, but her hypopituitarism—a rare condition that causes proportional dwarfism—makes her look like a child. The body of the adoptee, a body of uncertain origin that harbors secrets and disguises itself with malicious intent, is thus identified as the source of horror unleashed on the unsuspecting family and community.

Orphan is not original in its use as a horror effect of the adoptee's visibly normal but noncompliant body, which is unsusceptible to socialization or rehabilitation. Like *The Bad Seed* and many other films of the "evil child" genre, *Orphan* relies on the uncanny affect evoked in the viewer by the body that does not comply with the representational "ideology of the physical" (Mitchell and Snyder 15). This ideology presumes correspondence between surface deformities and villainy. But this "generic convention capable of yield[ing] the pleasure of universal recognition" (15) is subverted when the body of a child, typically read as a reliable sign of innocence, powerlessness, and dependence, is portrayed as ridden with evil, manifested as the drive to stop at nothing in an attempt to manipulate the environment. While in *The Bad Seed* and *The Omen* such representational device is used quite straightforwardly—the bodies of little innocent-looking children carry "bad genes" that shape their psychopathic character no matter what their upbringing is—*Orphan* works through an intricate mistaken-identity plot built around a hidden physical disability that becomes a metaphor for the cultural anxiety over the adoptee's unknown origin. In doing this, the film explores cultural mechanisms that regulate (in)visibility of adoptive families within heterocoital cultures and, specifically, the practice of concealing the child's adoptive status by manipulating the perception of the adoptee's body. But it also reveals cultural perceptions of adoption as a form of disability that requires rehabilitation.[12] Rehabilitation in this context is understood as both physical, rooted in the histories of disabled children adopted from Eastern Europe, including those with hidden disabilities, and metaphorical, focused on aligning the adoptee's psyche and behavior with the adoptive culture's expectations for the kind of body an adoptee inhabits.

Imagery associated with the adoptee's body is commonly used across different types of adoption narratives as a way of exploring the meanings of secrecy in adoption. For instance, in the adoptee-point-of-view narratives—especially in the search and reunion narrative—the adoptee's body may be simultaneously a painful reminder of difference from the adoptive family and a welcome repository of genealogical knowledge that holds a promise of recovering the pre-adoption past and belonging with the birth family. This tension may be explored with the aim of challenging secrecy in adoption and revealing its harmful effects on an adoptee's psyche. The horror genre's engagement with the adoptee's body imagery, however, follows the logic of the narratives that reflect the adoptive culture's point of view. In such narratives, an adoptee's intersectionality, signaled by the body, may be portrayed as

12. The addition of the disability studies perspective to this discussion is motivated by Lisa Cartwright's observations about the prominence of the hidden disability rhetoric in Eastern European adoptions, the link Emily Hipchen (2104) establishes between adoption and disability in her discussion of birth mothers' memoirs as disability narratives, and the overall ubiquity of disability discourse consistently coupled with secrecy in adoption culture. Adoption in American culture has been consistently conceived of as rehabilitation, a process of normalizing and managing reproductive difference.

something that needs to be normalized in order to meet the larger culture's conditions for belonging. The normalization mechanisms do change over time, and we can see both secrecy and openness in representations of adoption in horror film. But we also see that the cultural demand for managing the adoptee's reproductive difference survives, even though the mechanisms get modified. While *The Bad Seed* and *The Omen* deal with fears around full secrecy about the adoptee's origins in a context similar to closed records adoption where the adoptee can pass for "one-of-us," *Orphan* engages with a more complex dynamic of adoptee origin disclosure, one characteristic of more recent understanding of transnational adoption, which necessitates the preservation of the adoptee's connection to their origins and pre-adoption past. The transnational adoptee's difference in such cases could be visibly anchored in the adoptee's body through rituals of keeping birth-culture and through a narrative of belonging that safely integrates the adoptees' biological, foreign origin into the adoptive family story. The body of the adoptee becomes a means of modulating, not erasing, the adoptee's difference.

Whether the child's otherness is accentuated or downplayed typically depends on the degree of racial matching between children and their adoptive parents. The correlation between similarity in racial features of parents and adopted children and the family's effort to sustain the adoptee's ethnocultural difference through active incorporation of birth culture in the family life, observed by Sara Dorow and by Heather Jacobson, is tightly tied to the ability of an adoptive family to reveal or conceal their adoptive status. For example, a significant number of adoptive parents of children from Russia and China understood their work of "culture keeping" as hedging against the adoptee's possible nonbelonging within larger communities (Jacobson 2008). Parents of Chinese adoptees stressed the now widely recognized importance of maintaining the adoptees' birth culture as part of their identity in order to facilitate their functioning in racialized American society. In contrast, many parents of children adopted from Russia were worried "that over-emphasizing their Russian heritage might create difficulties for their children as white, middle-class American children" (125). It is telling that the intersection of adoption and race leads to imagining the child's future as compliance with cultural formations specific to the child's race, without accommodation of their adoptive hybrid status. While minimizing the adoptee's difference for the sake of adoptive family unity, the family feels obligated to manage (amplify or reduce) this difference in a way that will prepare the child for recognizing and performing racialized reproductive protocols employed within the adoptive culture. The adoptee is expected to reproduce racial formations even as their adoption challenges them. The adoptee's known origin (a must in the open-adoption culture) thus produces its own set of anxieties that need to be managed by the adoptive culture in ways that assure its own reproduction through the reproductively (and often racially or ethnically) different bodies of adoptees.

In adoption horror, the change from secrecy to openness in adoption manifests in the transformation of the cultural anxiety over the hidden threat (unknown origin) into the fear of the known, managed threat (recognized cultivated origin) that can escape the control of the adoptive family at any time. The destabilizing effect of the adoptee's origin is thus distributed over the whole adoptive family, which is othered by the adoptee's reproductive difference and tasked with bringing the adoptee into the fold of American culture and family as "one of us." Since such normalization implies creating an identity perceived as different but nonthreatening by the larger culture, the fear of the full origin's return remains. Horror representations of adoption reflect the idea that given the lingering power of the American ideology of familial nation formation to reinscribe national, racial, and genealogical categories situated by birthright (Jerng 2010), American adoption works to signify the otherness of the adoptee no matter how "integrated" or racially similar they may be to the adoptive culture or family. The boundary separating the "foreign" and the "domestic," never allowed to be dissolved completely, serves to mitigate the perception of the disruptive power of the adoptee's origin (because a threat that is known can be managed), yet the cost of such safety is the constant awareness of possible disruption. This ambiguity is one of the driving forces of the adoption horror genre.

In plotting her deception, Esther responds to cultural mechanisms of dealing with her difference. She addresses the anxiety of the adoptive culture over the invisible difference of the same-race adoptee by styling her body in a way that signals transparency about her origin. Even though she might be able to pass for a member of a white American family, she chooses to keep her difference inscribed on her body. Though she has spent several years among English speakers, Esther speaks with a heavy Russian accent, and in general seems to make little effort to "blend in." She seems to reject any regular children's clothing different from her signature Victorian-style dresses. A picture-perfect "good girl," she often wears them with aprons. She never takes ribbons off from around her neck and wrists, which intensifies her "Victorian" look and moves a nun at the orphanage to exclaim: "She is such a princess!" Esther's insistence on emphasizing her difference seems to declare transparency—I am what I am. And even though her performance emphasizes her separateness from the family, it serves to strengthen her bond with them by ensuring her new kin that she has nothing to hide. The horror effect is achieved in the film when her body, which appears sufficiently marked by difference acceptable to the adoptive culture (ethnic, eccentric), is revealed to be a bearer of another kind of difference: a psychopathic adult passing as an innocent child. Each of the signs that help her performance is also a sign of the secrets that she keeps. The dresses work to conceal the parts of her body that may betray her real age, and the ribbons cover the scars left by restraints used by the mental hospital staff to subdue her violent behavior. The success of Esther's manipulations depends on her balancing the performance of her adoptive difference with manifested compliance to the affective "rules" of the adoptive family and culture. She is a "perfect child" in her emotional expressions and behavior—a performance that makes her visible reproductive difference nonthreatening and fools everyone. The terrifying effect of the revelation of Esther's "true nature" hinges on the fact that Esther's secret is not really hidden; it is written all over her body. And while the secret is, literally, in front of the family's and viewer's eyes all the time, her difference remains misread until the real story of her past comes to light.

Esther seems to engage in a peculiar version of what disability studies scholar Tobin Siebers calls "masquerade"—a concept he borrows from feminist and queer theories to describe a very specific form of passing by a disabled person that involves "claim[ing] disability as a version of itself rather than simply concealing it from view" (101). As Siebers explains, "masquerade represents an alternative method of managing social stigma through disguise" (102). Such "passing" involves not crossing over into the dominant social group, but, on the contrary, assuming an identity that is socially stigmatized or disadvantaged in a different way. Esther, whose condition shapes her body to look like a child's, chooses to pass as a child—a dependent identity socially inferior to that of an adult. She also chooses to maintain her grotesque foreignness and remain an unassimilated immigrant—a demonstrative "honest" refusal to pass as a typical white American girl. In doing that, she indulges the cultural expectation of maintaining connections to her birth culture and uses her adoptive difference to exercise a form of resistance to the "ideology of ability," according to which, "the more visible the disability, the greater chance that the disabled person will be repressed from the public view and forgotten" (103). She finds her way out of an institution and invisibility by "parading" her disability in her transnational adoptee impersonation—an expression of difference that is still more culturally acceptable than who—or what—she really is.

By doing this, Esther seems to challenge the understanding of the adoptees' incorporation into the American family, larger community, culture, and nation as akin to rehabilitation of people with disabilities. Rehabilitation is described by Henri-Jacques Stiker as driven by the goal of "making alterity disappear" by means of "identification, of making [the disabled body] identical" or at least approximate to the norm (qtd. in McRuer 118). According to McRuer, by its very nature, rehabilitation demands "integration into society as it is"; it "demands compliance or—more properly—makes noncompliance unthinkable" (112–13).[13] *Orphan,* as do narratives of disrupted Eastern European adoption, demonstrate that an encounter between adoption as rehabilitation philosophy and the *as if* ideology of American adoption produce cultural anxiety over anticipated compliance breaches by noncompliant bodies or bodies that only appear compliant. In Esther's case, rehabilitation means eventually assuming the identity of a white, upper-middle-class child and then adult. Her body is presented simultaneously as noncompliant in its expression of her adoptive status and yet moving toward compliance since the difference that Esther preserves as camouflage is within the range of acceptable expressions by a nine-year-old transnational adoptee. She is not perceived as resisting rehabilitation; her adoptive parents explain the right pronunciation of English words and consider her clothes choices a phase that should pass. In other words, she is perceived as still a *becoming-adult,* capable of eventually belonging and becoming part of the adoptive culture's futurity after her correct socialization. The horror is that she is already an adult who cannot be rehabilitated further to fully integrate into adoptive culture.

By hiding her disability in plain view, Esther is able to commit subversive acts of resistance that defy the rehabilitation and normalization project of adoption. These acts, albeit less obviously than killings, also gradually reveal her to the audience as a monster. She is adopted by the Colemans as a substitute for Kate's stillborn baby, Jessica, and is expected to heal the family's reproductive wound. Yet, she seems to resist the unspoken demand for such healing by signaling to others Kate's inability to reproduce, through her expressions of foreignness. The act of cutting baby Jessica's memorial roses is another act of rejection of her role as a substitute child. And ultimately, in the seduction scene, her coming-out-as-an-adult moment, Esther makes her pass at John by saying, "Let me take care of you"—a double entendre which could be heard as an erotic offer but also as her claim to being a caregiver, not a dependent. In the life of deception that she leads, she is enacting quite literally the perpetual cultural infantilization of the adoptee, and her disclosure to John is a way to resist the perpetual state of dependency and silence about her own desires.

13. The meaning of the adoptee's identity in the context of the rehabilitation project is cardinally different from the one employed by identity-based adult adoptees' movements. "Identity" in this sense signifies compliance and erasure of difference, identity-with-culture but not the celebration of "otherness" or of the possibility for resistance.

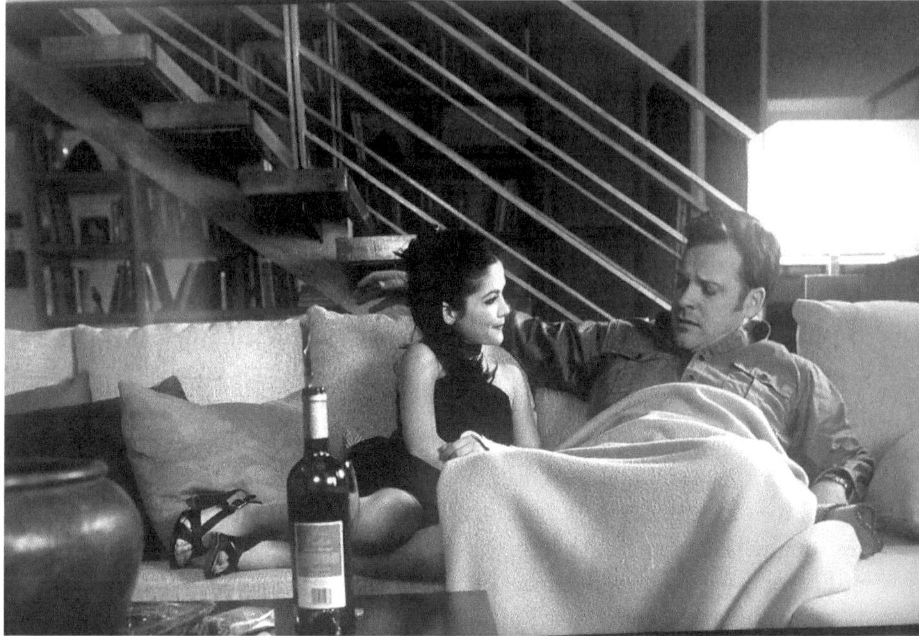

FIGURE 2.1. Ester seducing John in *Orphan*. Dark Castle Entertainment, 2009.

Even though her disorder facilitates her manipulation of caregivers, it is also a source of her frustrations. Her desires are incompatible with the kinship structure she is using to survive, and a disclosure of her adult status turns her into a monster that has to be banished from the family. The blurring of a clear moral boundary is a thrill heightened by plot sequencing that reveals Esther's true origins and murder history parallel to her seduction of and confrontation with John.

By making a pass at John (see figure 2.1), Esther reveals herself as what Julia Kristeva calls "the abject" and Margrit Shildrick the "monster"—a state of being that serves to consolidate the normal by representing that which is "ejected beyond the scope of the possible, the tolerable, the thinkable" (Kristeva 1). Esther is "all that must be excluded in order to secure the ideal of an untroubled social order" (Shildrick 3). But, as both Kristeva and Shildrick explain, the fear and disgust inspired by such a monster are not inspired by its deviance only but by the suggestion that such deviance is enmeshed with the normal, and the normal cannot be constituted without the "abject." Such interdependence produces fearsome hybridity—"the in-between, the ambiguous, the composite" (Kristeva 4), which, at the level of the body, underscores the "problematic ontology of a human being" (Shildrick 3) and, in the context of adoption, points to the anxiety about uncertain origins. Esther's childish body driven by adult sexuality is monstrous because it "does not respect borders, positions, rules" (Kristeva 4). And it is doubly abject because it is not openly amoral (which, according to Kristeva can even be respected) but "immoral, sinister, scheming and shady" (4). Esther appears to be one thing and turns out to be another; she is something that can never be squarely named the other in the child-adult binary. Therefore, she represents a greater threat than a known monster by "being [a monster that is] all too human" (Shildrick 3).

Esther is a sexual being with desires directed at the man who is culturally recognized as her father, and her attraction to him is a forbidden incestuous impulse that undermines the heterocoital order. By connecting origins and incest in a horrifying plot conflict, *Orphan* draws attention to yet another way the origins discourse functions to maintain the primacy of heterocoital family. In her study of genetic sexual attraction in adoption, Frances Latchford names incest as the "discourse [that] demarcates people as 'family' on the basis of biology" and "a test that delineates the boundaries of family in the modern Western context" (228). She connects the "idealization of biological ties over and above adoptive ties and the prohibition against incest" as "two sides of the same coin" that "work together to uphold the bio-genealogical imperative as the modern Western truth of family" (224). In *Orphan*, Esther's sexual desire for John challenges the viewer's understanding of their relationship as *real* kinship and achieves two goals. On the one hand, the viewers are invited to consider with fear and disgust the possibility of incest and reconfirm their aversion toward it; on the other hand, they may see that what is happening between Esther and John is not quite incest by definition and, since such dubious situation seems to be the product of adoption, the viewers renew their commitment to heterocoital family and known origin. Nontraditional kinship is confirmed as unsafe. The horror of the situation for the viewer lies both in seeing a child (visible age) make sexual advances and a child (conventionally read as a biological relative) make sexual advances at her father. Esther is a monster because she cannot experience and express her desire and affect according to acceptable cultural scripts that regulate relationships between members of a family. She cannot be a part of a family, neither from a commonsensical nor from a psychoanalytical perspective: she is horrible in her breaking of heterocoital taboos. But the very special horror here is that, given the lack of biological ties to the adoptive family and her actual age, it is possible to think that she is not *really* (read: by heterocoital logic) breaking any rules.

This horrifying ambiguity is a consequence of the cultural commitment to as-ifness of the adoptive family—in other words, its perpetual, unresolved, hybrid, and so, "monstrous" status, which is called upon to shore up the value of the heterocoital family. While, in the case of a heterocoital family, the rule would be unambiguous—thou shall not desire your blood relative—Esther's situation, when it comes to light, raises questions about this rule. Dealing with Esther thus is a matter of confirming the boundaries of what family *is* in a situation where biology cannot be leaned on as an immutable, and thus unquestionable, buttress of morality. Her attempt to disable Kate and seduce John, the photos of her other adoptive fathers she keeps, and the concealed erotic drawings on the walls of her bedroom show that she wants a different role in this or any other family she has been with as an adoptee; she is looking to be a wife, not a child (or—worse yet—both a wife and a child). But her condition, as long as it is concealed, only allows her entry into a family structure as a child—a scenario in which her sexuality is read as incestuous and destructive to the family. The film is not really concerned with an exploration of Esther's motivations and suffering, but it lets us know quite clearly that a life in which Esther's hypopituitarism is acknowledged and in which she gains entry into the heterocoital order as a wife or a mother is unimaginable. *Orphan* denies the adoptee the status of a link in a genealogical chain as it couples the impossibility of disabled sexuality with common cultural imaginings of adoptees as perennial children whose adult identities beyond the adoptive family structure "excee[d] a culture's predictive capacities" in the way disability does (Mitchell and Snyder 3).

Within the logic of the film, Esther does not seem to have a life path that could involve both a disclosure of her disability (and her pre-adoption past) and an acceptance into the traditional family structure, which insists on able-bodied sexuality capable of reproduction. In a culture where reproductive "sex and human ability are both ideologically and inextricably linked," according to Siebers, "people with disabilities" have to contend with a widespread cultural assumption "that they cannot, will not, or should not contribute to the future of the human race" (140). It is not surprising then that even though Esther is technically an adoptee, the film insists on calling her an "orphan"—a concept different in its implications from the cultural understanding of the adoptee.[14] While the adoptee is "one of us," even if "not quite," the orphan is "an outsider, a body without family ties to the community, a foreigner" (Peters 6). In that sense, Esther—an adoptee incapable of forging the right kind of family bonds—remains an orphan for the duration of the film. In her study of orphan characters in Victorian literature, Laura Peters observes that "the orphan, as one who embodie[s] the loss of the family, [comes] to

14. David Smolin draws a theological distinction between adoptees and orphans, for example. Laura Peters, discussed here, analyzes the difference between them in literary representations.

represent a dangerous threat" to the integrity of the family; as a consequence, in literary plots involving an orphan, the family may "reaffir[m] itself through the expulsion of this threatening difference" (2). In horror, the impossibility to "confidently narrate [such characters'] future" (Mitchell and Snyder 3), typically effects death or some other form of obliteration. *Orphan* ends with Kate fighting and killing Esther—with a little help from Max—at the pond by the house. Esther's death in the pond, where Max almost drowned several months earlier due to neglect while Kate was abusing alcohol, confirms the "right" family configuration and signals which bodies are considered preferable for continuation and reproduction within a family structure. The scene arrests the viewers' imagination at the point where it would be possible to envision a culture that accommodates Esther's difference. By killing Esther, Kate kills Esther's chance to enter the heterocoital order as an adult.

Orphan's ending also suggests a certain hierarchy of disability, in which Max's deafness and Kate's alcoholism are ranked as more socially acceptable than the deceptive disability which marks Esther's body as nonreproductive and undermines her ability for affective exchanges acceptable in a middle-class American family. The difference between disabilities lies in the degrees of their visibility, manageability, and impact on affective performance. While Max's deafness is relatively apparent and is managed within the family environment and school by means of sign language and hearing aids, and while Kate's alcoholism is well known to people close to her and has been under control, Esther's disabilities are unknown, invisible, or at least not immediately identifiable, and—what is worse—they make her incapable of affect that would assure her belonging within the family and the community. She can act as a well-behaved child, but ultimately the performance falls apart when her goals and desires become apparent and tear the social fabric apart. *Orphan* suggests that disabilities that are known, contained, and managed within the family may be more acceptable than those that stubbornly resist rehabilitation or those that remain invisible yet threatening. It also suggests that disabilities that do not interfere with affect that holds a family together are acceptable, while affective disorders are perceived as threats. The condition of belonging is the adoptee's ability to experience and perform their affective states in the ways that confirm their loyalty to the adoptive culture and family. The responsibility for fostering such affect in an adopted child and constructing their difference as nonthreatening to the larger culture has rested mostly on the adoptive family, which—historically—has served as a rehabilitative space.

The similarity between this role of the adoptive family and disability discourses prompts us to look at adoption as a form of rehabilitation within the framework of Robert McRuer's analysis of the American family as an institution functioning to reproduce able-bodied heterosexuality. McRuer claims that at the turn of the twentieth century, following the strengthening of capitalism, the idea of the heterosexual able-bodied "orderly, managed home" emerged as an antithesis to "the (perceived) unruly, disorderly homes of the poor, people of color, and (especially) immigrants" (91). One of the main functions of such home was reproduction of disciplined, able bodies capable of physiological and psychological self-control—a project that often went hand in hand with normalizing cultural, ethnic, and racial differences. McRuer draws a suggestive connection between able-bodiedness and racialization as a form of social engineering, quoting Henrietta Goodrich, a "domestic science expert" from the beginning of the twentieth century: "It was, in fact, the home (that is, the white, middle-class home), 'brought into harmony with industrial conditions and social ideals' in the larger world, that would forestall what Theodore Roosevelt and others called 'race suicide'" (91). Such assessment of the role of the family in American culture, as an institution responsible for integrating racial, cultural, and ethnic difference into the American nation, aligns with Julie Berebitsky's observations on the role of adoptive families in "rescuing" the American nation from the threats of immigration by turning young immigrants into rehabilitated, assimilated Americanized children (84). Whether transnational adoption is positioned as rescue or—more recently—as an exchange that benefits both parent and child, it is imagined in American culture as adoptees' assimilation into American family, community, and larger culture through affective rehabilitation.

Narratives of same-race Eastern European adoptions often demonstrate that an important aspect of managing transnational adoptees' reproductive difference has been fostering their compliance with class-inflected affective scripts, specifically, the middle-class ideal of the sentimental, unproductive child. This concept, according to Viviana Zelizer, emerged at the end of the nineteenth and the beginning of twentieth centuries due to the changing role of the family as a site of consumption and the emergence of American middle class. Since social "concern has moved from fitting bodies for factory production to pursuing the demands of the consumer society" (Barnes and Mercer 84), the child now acquires emotional value contingent upon their participation in the exchange of affect within the family, and the family acquires an additional responsibility of reproducing bodies with the capacity for the right kind of affect. Horror films like *Orphan* show, as do disrupted adoptions, that an adoptee's inability to control and perform appropriate and appropriately addressed emotions precludes the adoptee from membership in a family or community unified by a certain protocol of affective exchanges. Such a breakdown, which typically drives a horror film plot, draws attention to the emotional labor of children, and adoptees in particular, that culture may demand as a means to maintaining socially valued kinship structures. An adoption situation makes the family's emotional labor that goes into affective performances and exchanges more obvious than those of the heterocoital family. For example, the adoptee's perceived failure to experience and express gratitude to the adoptive family, community, and nation may be perceived as disloyal, deviant, and a threat to unity, since a child's gratitude to their parents is culturally construed as a given, even though this is not always the case in heterocoital families. The task of disciplining the adoptee's affect, in turn, disciplines the affective exchanges of the adoptive family as a whole. The capacity to experience and channel socially acceptable affect that supports cultural primacy of the heterocoital family is a condition of social inclusion that has to be met by all family members. The figure of the "unsalvageable adoptee" in horror narratives thus represents also the horror of the adoptive family's inability to rehabilitate the adopted child fully, its becoming corrupted and consumed by the adoptee's difference, and thus its failure to reproduce the values associated with heterocoital kinship.

In order to "save" the sociocultural value of adoptive family as a culturally acceptable imitation of heterocoital family, *Orphan* connects the impairment of affect to the body of the adoptee, which makes the impairment intractable and beyond any possible interventions available to the normative nuclear family. Esther's psychopathic personality is loosely associated with her physical, incurable condition by the representational logic of the film, even though cause-effect relationships between hypopituitarism and psychopathology are not a given. The unsalvageable adoptee is relegated, then, to the category of orphans—emotionally unattached strangers: unknown, unhomely, and uncanny, existing outside kinship. The expulsion from the family of the adoptee incapable of performing required scripts of white, middle-class, able-bodied childhood, which we see in *Orphan,* is a plot turn that reaffirms the normative configuration of the heterocoital family by placing the orphan, a scapegoat of sorts, outside the familial structure. The ending of *Orphan* follows the formula in which the discovery and confirmation of the monster results in the killing of the monster. During their fight at the pond, Kate explicitly reinscribes Esther's orphanhood by ignoring her pleas to be saved, pushing her underwater, and saying, "I am not your fucking mommy!" This act of refusal to protect Esther's well-being and life makes Kate's disavowal of the mother-child bond final, and Kate's choice to save Max instead reaffirms heterocoital family as a guarantor of protection against the evil.

Yet, orphans are "not truly outside the narrative of domesticity," according to Peters, who claims that "the orphan is not a foreign invading threat but is actually produced by and hence is an essential component of the family itself" (22)—a variation on Kristeva's abject and Shildrick's monster. Drawing on the analogy that appears in Freud's essay "The Uncanny," Peters compares an orphan to "a hidden spring," a secret, which lies under a pond—the family—and "might reappear at any moment . . . thus making the family both untrustworthy and unstable" (22). Peters's comparison encapsulates the nature of tensions that arise from understanding adoption as rehabilitation. According to McRuer's reading of Stiker, "rehabilitation marks the appearance of a culture that attempts to complete the act of identification, of making identical" (113). The socially acceptable identity of the rehabilitated adoptee, then, should be more concerned with the erasure of difference than its assertion. And such successful rehabilitation may produce adoptees who, on their own, can pass as individuals heterocoitally produced by their adoptive parents. Yet, for the adoptees themselves, and as long as the adoptee is within the adoptive family structure, the erasure of difference can never become complete. The as-if philosophy of adoption insists only on approximation to the norm: the adoptee has to be "one of us" but still a little bit of an orphan. In other words, the adoptee's reproductive difference has to be somehow preserved even if it is concealed. The preserved difference can only be translated into identifications continuous with the ones already existent in the adoptive culture, since "the ideology of rehabilitation can only comprehend 'integration' according to its own terms" (92). The adoptee is expected to become "transparent" and known on the adoptive culture's terms—a process which conceals one truth as it creates another. But the adoptee's past and origin remain the hidden springs, always ready to send ripples across the surface of the family pond.

In adoption horror that essentializes the adoptee's abnormal affect, that is, portrays it as originating in the body and genetics, the solution to the threat of such a hidden spring is typically the killing of the evil adoptee. The adoptee's body is seen as a conduit for evil due to its faulty genetics, so it has to be destroyed. Such portrayals of "nature" as persistently manifesting itself in the adoptee's affect and behavior affirm the primacy of heterocoital kinship in *Orphan*. This primacy is also confirmed by the ultimate survival of the adoptive family, which, following the purge of the monster, ceases to be adoptive and is restored to its heterocoital configuration. In adoption horror where the source of the adoptee's wickedness is unhealed early childhood trauma, adoptive families may survive the challenges presented by the disturbed adoptee, but the hidden threat to family and community integrity remains lurking behind the facade of normalcy. In the made-evil adoptee narratives, the parents' (typically adoptive mothers') enduring loyalty to their children is portrayed as a dubious happy ending. Such mother figures may be cast as both heroic and foolish in their loyalty to children who are still potentially destructive to the community. The origin of the adoptee may become known, but the adoptee's "true nature" remains ambiguous, and the anxiety about their loyalty and belonging remains unresolved. The decision of the adoptive parents to remain loyal to the adopted child is portrayed as precarious, and the adoptive family may be portrayed as "othered" by its reintegration of a seemingly rehabilitated adoptee. Overall, in horror films, the adoptive family does not seem able to win: if it saves itself and the community by killing the adoptee, it ceases to exist as an adoptive family; if it remains loyal to the adoptee while the adoptee's goodness is in question, it is othered since it fails in its responsibility to socialize the adopted child into a stable guarantor of uninterrupted futurity for community, nation, and humanity. *Luce* (2019), a film that unfolds according to this evil-by-trauma scenario, follows its narrative and affective logics as it explores the project of rehabilitating an adoptee traumatized by having been a child soldier.

Luce, a film by Julius Onah based on a 2013 play by J. C. Lee, is not a classical horror film; it has been commonly classified as a thriller or thriller-drama. Yet, this film deals with the subject matter of adoption according to the representational logic of an adoption horror film. The cultural understanding of the adoptee as "the hidden spring" gives *Luce* its thrill. It activates the viewers' anxiety over the adoptee's capacity for belonging in the adoptive culture and follows the basic conflict of the adoption horror film: a visibly normal and exemplary adoptee exhibits malicious behavior and affect that are beyond the control of the adoptive family and community. *Luce* makes an interesting case because it shifts the perspective, even if it is only a little bit, toward the adoptee's point of view, and this shift gives the film a meta aspect that invites the viewer to consider causes of the adoptee's behavior in a more complex way. Instead of locating the reasons for the adoptee's behavior wholly in the past, *Luce* explores how the process of adaptation to and surviving in the adoptive family and culture contributes to the lack of social trust in the adoptee. Unlike a typical horror film, where the adoptee may be a monster or a traumatized child without complex interiority, *Luce* gives the audience some access to the thoughts and feelings of its main character, a former child soldier from Eritrea and a high school senior adopted by a white American couple. The viewer knows just enough to speculate about possible reasons for his struggles with rehabilitation. The adoptee of *Luce* is different and, perhaps, more anxiety-inducing because he is smarter and more calculating than a typical psychopathic adoptee of the horror genre. He is also more "normal" and thus capable of activating the viewers' sympathy during the confirmation stage of the "complex discovery plot" that serves to prove the monster's wickedness (Carroll 99). The viewer is not in the position of knowing more about Luce than other characters do and thus of being any more certain of his evil or innocence. In fact, most of *Luce*'s action is stuck at the confirmation stage; its plot does not move into a definitive confirmation of a monster's evil nature followed by an open confrontation and banishment. Luce's malice is never fully confirmed, yet, in the complex game of deception staged in the film, the viewer is never sure whether he is an innocent either. The tension is not completely resolved by the ending, because the adoptee's allegiance to his family, community, and nation remains ambiguous. The film continues to play with the viewers by inviting them to decide when and whether the adoptee's affect and loyalty are genuine.

Like Luce's adoptive parents and his school, the audience is pulled into figuring out how Luce feels about what he does in order to understand if he can be trusted. The expert acting by Kevin Harrison Jr., who plays Luce, serves this project well: expressions of his face, often emphasized by close-ups, give the audience clues about what he might be feeling and thinking. When his facial expressions are at odds with the viewer's expectations of appropriate affect or when they are signaling that the adoptee is lying about his genuine feelings, the anxiety over his presence within the adoptive family and community is heightened. But the expressions also reveal emotional struggles experienced by Luce, which foster the viewers' sympathy. The ambiguity about Luce's loyalties is also created by the sequencing of plot reversals that disrupt the viewer's emotional stances toward the adoptee: just when the audience may side with Luce, he is doing something that puts his moral character in question. A new plot twist may redeem him by revealing further motivation behind his actions, but not for long. Ultimately, even though *Luce* treats the subject of adoption with more complexity than a typical adoption horror film might, it still ends on a note that resonates with endings of horror films in which the adoptee, reabsorbed by the adoptive family, remains "the hidden spring" and his violent past a constant source of anxiety.

Post-adoption Luce is a star student, an example for the whole school. He is groomed by his history of government teacher, Ms. Wilson (Octavia Spencer), for an Ivy League school. His parents, the Edgars (Tim Roth and Naomi Watts), who have spent a great deal of resources on his therapy and integration into their white middle-class family, consider his rehabilitation a success. Amy Edgar is especially attached to the outcome of her committed effort to earn Luce's trust and establish an emotionally genuine relationship with him. While the details of his violent past are never discussed openly and never seem to be understood fully by his parents or Wilson, his pre-adoption experience remains constitutive to his identity and belonging in his adoptive family, community, and country. The ways in which his past is activated range from underscoring his present successes as extraordinary to perceiving him as a ticking time bomb that is capable of unleashing violence on his community. This ambiguity is set in motion by the sequence of the opening scenes.

A school locker is the first thing we see as the film begins. The music is eerie, and, together with a tracking shot that zeroes in on the locker door, it prompts anxious anticipation of discovering what is inside. We do not see whose locker this is, which adds to the anxiety and foreshadows the events that structure the film's conflict. The door is opened by an anonymous hand that adds to the locker's innocuous contents (books and a water bottle) a mysterious brown bag. It is revealed later that the locker is Luce's, and the bag holds dangerous fireworks. They are eventually discovered by Wilson, and Luce becomes a suspect, but his connection to the fireworks is assumed, not proven, because Luce's whole running team share each other's lockers. Wilson searches Luce's locker after he submits an assignment in her class—a paper in the voice of a famous political figure. He chooses Frantz Fanon and draws on ideas from "Concerning Violence," which Wilson takes as a sign of the return of his own violent tendencies. The opening locker scene is cut to an image of the empty school and then to the assembly hall where Luce, a brilliant speaker, is giving a speech to honor academic achievements of his fellow students. He acknowledges parents, without whom students, he says, "would be troops unprepared for the battles ahead of us." The metaphor seems innocent enough at first, but once the conflict between Luce and Wilson and Luce's origin become known to the viewer, this sequencing of scenes comes across as foreboding and contributes to the thrills of the plot. The opening scenes are shot with darkened lighting that casts everything in blue-gray cold tones—a contrast to Luce's uplifting words and facial expressions with which he expertly calibrates the emotional impact of his speech. He thanks teachers and parents "for helping us become who we were meant to be"—another phrase that carries ambiguous meaning: he might be speaking about reaching one's full potential or he might be suggesting that there is a mold everyone has to fit. Thus, without naming the conflict of the film explicitly, the opening sequence foreshadows Luce's struggle with trying to be who his parents and teacher want him to be and dealing privately with the inner turmoil caused by such disciplining of his affect and behavior.

In a brief conversation between Luce, Wilson, and his parents after the school assembly and on the ride home, it becomes clear that the relationship between Luce and Wilson is tense, even though it remains civil on the surface. A scene in Wilson's classroom further clarifies this tension. During a class on race and American law, Wilson is cruel to Deshaun Meeks, a Black student.

She disciplines him sternly, publicly humiliating him for looking at his phone. Wilson compares Deshaun to a white female student who is also checking her phone and says that for her the knowledge of American law is "incidental," but for him it could be "a matter of life and death." This incident foreshadows the reason for the conflict between her and Luce. He sees how the way she understands experiences of other people lacks complexity, leaning toward stereotyping and tokenism. In his own relationship with Wilson, he often experiences her expectations for him as a burden, a demand to be perfect, and a responsibility he did not ask for. He sees her as turning him into her variation on the "talented tenth" (Du Bois 31), and he resists the distinction she draws between him and Deshaun. In addition to sympathizing with Deshaun and wanting justice for him, Luce is sensing that failure to uphold his image may turn him, too, into a lost cause in Wilson's eyes. After Wilson reprimands Deshaun, the camera pulls back to show that Luce's gaze is locked with hers. Luce turns away first, and we can see his face—lost, resigned, his gaze following Wilson as she walks back to the front of the classroom. The camera stays on Luce, who looks back at Deshaun, taking in his dejection after the public humiliation. After class, Luce tries to talk to Deshaun, but Deshaun walks away. Luce gives Ms. Wilson a look of reproach, but she stares him down, and Luce loses this silent power struggle. Later, it is revealed that Wilson was instrumental to kicking Deshaun off the running team for smoking pot, and that Luce decides to "set things right" for Deshaun, who is demoralized and becoming engaged with the group of students who may be dealing drugs. Throughout the film, Luce skillfully manipulates Wilson, using his parents, the school principal, and his classmates in order to punish her both for ruining Deshaun's life and for not truly seeing him.

Another trigger for Luce's manipulation is a breach of trust between him and his parents caused by the way Wilson handles the incident with fireworks. She invites Amy Edgar to a parent-teacher conference to discuss Luce's paper written in the voice of Frantz Fanon. In this conversation, the viewers learn for the first time about Luce's "context," as Wilson puts it. She starts the conversation by stating that the school "cares a great deal about his success" and that it must have been hard for Amy and Peter, given Luce's "background," to successfully parent in this situation. Wilson mentions language and culture shock as challenges, but her hesitations signal that she is choosing her language carefully and is also implying something else. She does not seem to remember where Luce is from originally, and Amy has to prompt her with the name "Eritrea" when Wilson begins to talk about Luce's coming from a "war zone." Luce's past is invoked by Wilson to justify her concern over Luce's choice to write his paper in the voice of Frantz Fanon, whom she describes to

Amy, unfamiliar with his work, as a revolutionary who advocated violence as a way to liberate the colonized from the colonizer. The scene of Wilson handing Luce's essay to Amy is cut to Luce walking to the gym shower. His face has a hard look, like there is too much to bear—a stark contrast to his usual smile. The camera follows him to the shower, he turns sideways, exhales, and draws the curtain. Such intercutting directs the viewer's attention to Luce's suppressed rage and fatigue from the rehabilitation process, which demands he hide feelings that may undermine its success. The attention is also drawn to Wilson's attempt to impose her understanding of Luce onto Amy, thus putting in question the social success Amy is so proud of—her rehabilitation of the troubled adopted son.

The scene cuts back to Amy and Wilson, and their discussion of Luce's essay reveals the impact of Luce's past on his identity, family, and community as well as the ways in which his past is handled to meet the conditions of his belonging in the adoptive culture. After Wilson gives Amy her version of who Fanon is, Amy, surprised, asks, "You teach this?" Wilson replies, "I don't," with emphasis that makes Fanon seem like a forbidden subject. Their discussion of Luce's use of Fanon seems to have a narrow understanding of Fanon—literal, with no attention to the historical context of colonization that is also a part of Luce's "context." At the same time, the premise of the assignment (to *pretend* to be writing as a historical figure) is forgotten, and Wilson takes Luce's choice of this voice as a literal expression of his views. Wilson justifies searching Luce's locker by claiming that in his paper, Luce made a call "to gun down those you disagree with." Her handling of the situation shows that she acknowledges Luce's past but refuses to engage with its complexity and to see Luce as a transnational adoptee whose life has been shaped as much by colonialism and immigration experience as by the American system of race relationships. Wilson, a representative voice of Luce's adoptive community, accepts him on condition he complies with her vision of him as a successful African American man. His pre-adoption past is thus de-emphasized as constitutive of his identity and is seen as just an obstacle he was able to overcome through hard work with the help of the adults. A narrow understanding of his history is activated only as an explanation for cracks in his image, and his foreignness is invoked as a way of shifting responsibility for such cracks away from the adoptive community.

While Luce's successes are recognized and appreciated, there is a lingering suspicion that he, a transnational adoptee and a former child soldier, may have remained "who he is" no matter how rehabilitated he can seem. In response to Wilson's doubts about the outcomes of Luce's "treatment" and the extent of his "adjustment," Amy insists that Luce went through recovery and "showed no signs of—" and that violence that he may have "experienced or inflicted" was "processed." Luce understands this expectation and tries to meet it, but he experiences trying to be as perfect as the adults want him to be as a source of emotional suffering that goes unnoticed by others. There are several moments in the film when Luce directly communicates his feelings to the adults. On one occasion, he tells Amy plainly that she cannot understand how hard he works to "keep it together" and that he can't be perfect. He rejects the all-or-nothing approach of Wilson and says that Wilson is talking about everyone as a symbol. Luce thinks that in her view, students "exist to confirm the world is the way she sees it" and that his role in her world is that of "a fucking poster boy," a "Black kid who overcame his tragic past, the example of why America works," a token, well-adjusted immigrant and an African American man, who lives to prove that Black success is possible in America. He refuses to see a difference between stereotypes and tokens, and when Amy says that one comes with benefits, he replies, "What you'd call a benefit, I'd call a responsibility I didn't ask for."

His resistance to the expectations of the adults is a resistance to being socialized into assuming a character, a voice, and an affective stance demanded by the community in order to maintain its own sense of safety. While Amy questions Wilson's actions and accusations and ultimately chooses to trust Luce, even though she cannot fully understand him, she still encourages him to maintain this character and voice, in order to "protect" him. She never explains from whom, but her comment invokes the complex interplay of performances imposed on Black men to signal their being "safe" for the others, even though they are not safe themselves. Luce believes that the adults who think of protecting him are really protecting "the idea" of him while at the same time "waiting for [him] to confirm this thing that no one wants to say out loud." He is "trying so hard not to be that," but he feels like he is fighting a losing battle and only gets to be a saint or a monster. Luce counters the claims that his image is for his own protection with "What if you are part of what you are protecting me from?" He challenges Amy's belief that she has always accepted him "for whoever you are" and demands that he be seen and known. But beyond that, he demands that his parents and community begin to know themselves. His manipulation pushes them to engage with the fact that he may be capable of violence (the fireworks story ends with Wilson's desk being blown up one night) but also to see what damage might be done to family and community ties if fears of and reasons for such fears are not discussed openly.

Luce recognizes himself as a site of struggle over which culture and what futurity his body is going to reproduce. This struggle is not openly recognized by his adoptive parents and community, yet it is made visible to the viewers through shots and scenes where they can see Luce's emotional expressions at the times when he doesn't think he is being observed. The guidance Luce receives from adults and their relationships is haunted by the specters of (post) colonial and uncomfortable Blackness, but, as he observes, they are never named "out loud," much less consciously unpacked and processed. He has to contend on his own with layers of his history and Blackness that go beyond the African American context the adults have in mind. Wilson is grounding him in African American history, which he is now a part of, and sees him as a sign of Du Boisean futurity for Black Americans—one of the "exceptional men" that could save the race (Du Bois 33). But her vision excludes diasporic dimensions of his identity (except for the assimilated immigrant), and his success on her terms seems also to necessitate an erasure of the state of being and becoming that Deshaun represents. The Edgars work hard on his rehabilitation and his class status, which can protect him from the dangers a Black man faces in America. In aiming to make Luce, a Black transnational adoptee, "one of us," the adoptive parents and community "edit" his origin and read his Black body as genealogically connecting him to a narrow understanding of African American history. The complexity of his origin, which may also tie him to abject violence and expressions of Blackness that are not acceptable to his community, becomes the ever-present "monster" that has to be silenced and controlled, first of all by Luce himself. Yet, the monster is never going away and is called upon to explain lapses in Luce's perfect conduct. In this way, American culture "knows" Luce without truly understanding him. Such an assimilation process is conditioned by the cultural understanding of heterocoital origin and culture as inevitably linked and heterocoital reproduction as having predictive capacity for futurity. This assumed link between heterocoital reproduction and the transfer of culture is also present in the reading of the film by Odie Henderson, who calls Luce and Wilson "two Black people with different ideas about how America sees them, and how their *birth origins* shape their perceptions" (emphasis mine). Such reading draws due attention to Luce's context, yet the impact of adoption experience on "perceptions" needs to be further probed, since neither the neat division of cultural allegiances by origin nor an erasure of the cultural meaning of genealogical origin can give access to Luce's hybrid experience as a Black transnational, transracial adoptee in the US and an African American young man.

Luce's manipulations and questionable actions can be perceived as invitations to engage with the complexity of his context. But these attempts to make himself known are perceived by adults as subversive and threatening. When Luce is confronted by Amy about the contents of his paper, he asks whether she really had read it, implying that she and Wilson do not understand Fanon beyond the cliché image of a violent revolutionary. As a political psychologist interested in the effects of colonialism on the psyches of the colonizers and colonized, Fanon provides a certain context for understanding what happened to Luce in the first ten years of his life in Eritrea and, later, post-adoption. By choosing Fanon's voice for his assignment, Luce may be signaling the importance of his past to his present experience and inviting his parents and educators to engage with the complexities of his trauma and the emotional work he has to do to manage it for the sake of belonging in his adoptive family and community. But Wilson balks at Fanon's mentioning and immediately invokes the concern about Luce's violent tendencies, while Amy is trying to dismiss the paper as a pretend exercise that has no bearing on Luce's real ideas and feelings. Instead, Amy shifts the focus to his success at rehabilitation, which is a kind of denial that Luce's past is alive and operative in how he is. Their different reactions notwithstanding, both Wilson's and Amy's approaches are directed at assuring the adoptee's loyalty to the adoptive community. Both expect and understand violence as Luce's noncompliance with the implicit rules of belonging in the adoptive culture and a regression to his old trauma state (i.e., regression to pre-adoption affective anchors and attachments); his rage can be only understood by them as out-of-control affect and a breach in attachment to the adoptive family and community, not an emotion that Luce is consciously managing in the process of meeting the conditions of belonging. In this context, Luce's chosen way of resistance to the pressures of rehabilitation and assimilation—guerrilla-style manipulation, not Fanon's direct violence—is a shift adults struggle to recognize and directly respond to because they have a limited understanding of Luce's past and present states, as well as of Fanon's ideas. With his manipulation, Luce shows that Wilson and his parents do not understand him, just as they don't understand Fanon or themselves.

In "Concerning Violence," Fanon draws a distinction between the kinds of power exercised in the metropoles in contrast with the colonies—the "soft" discipline of capitalist societies is different from the violent colonial oppression:

> The colonized world is a world cut in two. The dividing line, the frontiers are shown by barracks and police stations. In the colonies it is the policeman and the soldier who are the official, instituted go-betweens, the spokesmen of the settler and his rule of oppression. In capitalist societies the educational system, whether lay or clerical, the structure of moral reflexes handed down from father to son, the exemplary honesty of workers who are given a medal after fifty years of good and loyal service, and the affection that springs from

> harmonious relations and good behavior—all these aesthetic expressions of respect for the established order serve to create around the exploited person an atmosphere of submission and of inhibition which lightens the task of policing considerably. (38)

Luce revolts against the discipline of the soft power that takes him up into the adoptive history, without an acknowledgment of his own, and tries to mold him into a figure palatable to the adoptive culture. He revolts against the discipline of affect as an invisible form of violence that blocks expressions of his rage: the rage of a Black man turned into a token and of an adoptee who is expected to feel grateful and whose full experience, and especially the cost of his success, is not understood and not fully shared by the community he has been made a part of. He has become a bearer of the adoptive history and a conduit of its culture, but the adoptive community has not become a bearer of his history. By choosing Fanon, he may also be suggesting that, soft power notwithstanding, there is a violent dividing line that structures his past and present experiences and that insists on bracketing out any expressions of self that are not consistent with the current image of a successful young African American man. Luce's past remains behind the line, suppressed, invoked only as an explanation of his failure to present as someone who the community wants him to be. In other words, his hybridity is denied its full expression.

As a transnational and transracial adoptee, an immigrant from Africa, Luce is pulled into American racial discourses without acknowledgment of how his history may engage with American history beyond the cliché narratives of model immigrant or model African American man. Sandra Patton (2000) observes that Black transracial adoptees have access to "systems of racial meaning" different from what Black children raised in African American communities have (11). In addition, *Luce* suggests that Black transnational adoptees face their own clash of racial meanings, similar yet different from those of Black immigrants to the United Sates, whose "understandings [have been] forged outside the national social formation of the United States" (Hintzen and Rahier 4). Luce's reckoning with the system of racial meanings that mediate his relationship with his parents, Wilson, and larger culture brings to mind the "the politics of deconstruction" (3) described by Hintzen and Rahier as an effect of the Black diaspora's presence in American culture. They write that such politics can "be deployed as much against the politics of blackness as it is against white racial authority (even though the former is itself deployed against the latter)" (4). Under such conditions, the narratives constitutive to Luce's identity cannot all fully converge to hybridize it; the narratives are activated, depending on the context, to signal Luce's belonging or non-belonging. This kind of hybridity is understood as shape-shifting and code-switching rather than a qualitatively new, truly hybrid subject position that is in itself a recognized cultural formation that may challenge identifications based on cultural scripts imposed on the adoptee. Adoption literature indeed shows that the hybridity of the transnational and transracial adoptee, which is often perceived as the freedom to navigate multiple social contexts, is not quite borne out by an adopted person's experience.[15]

Transnational, transracial adoptees are often perceived as having two identities that they can switch on and off depending on the context, without taking into account the personal costs for the adopted person who may not feel completely "at home" in any context except among adopted persons like themselves. The adoptee is expected to manage their connection to the birth culture by participating in rituals, going back to reconnect, and being an expert on the culture of their origin, but the condition of their belonging in the adoptive culture is the ability to "turn off" the foreignness and participate in and bear the system of racial meanings of the adoptive culture. Writing on transracial adoption, Sandra Patton (2000) says that adoptees' "identities argue for a recognition of the hybridity of identity" (14), a new way of being or cultural space that can be shared with and recognized by the adoptive culture. Transracial (and transnational) adoptees may feel like they "constitute [their] own race or ethnicity, or even belong to a separate ontological category of humans" (6). For Luce, as it may be for other transnational transracial adoptees, a cultural recognition of his truly hybrid subject position is out of reach. Ironically, only Luce's oblivious white friend Orlicki, who understands Luce as *one of a kind* (albeit in his own way)—"You are not Black. You are Luce," he says—comes close to recognizing the position Luce may feel like he is occupying.

While Luce seems socially connected across racial and class lines within his friend circle, and he enjoys mentorship of both white and Black authority figures—which is to say, he is moving across contexts with ease—still, whenever the film gives the viewer access to Luce's genuine affect, he is alone, and he isn't smiling. Luce's preparation for the graduation speech is a storyline that allows us to look beyond constant guessing about his noble or malicious

15. For example, Trenka writes about the inability to connect to Asian American student groups in school, and Eleana Kim (2010) writes about Korean adoptees interpellated by the Korean government as "global ambassadors" of Korea, effectively imagining the Korean transnational adoptee as a Korean and bracketing out adoptive experience. Patton (2000) also points out that identities of transracial adoptees "are often discussed in monolithic terms in the public discourse about transracial adoption, as if they develop either a White *or* a Black cultural identity" (11).

motivations and gives the viewer a glimpse of what could be his genuine feelings. When Luce practices his speech, alone, he opens with "I came to America, to this school, and I found myself." He flashes a smile that looks obviously overwrought. He follows with an anecdote about how Amy could not pronounce his original name and Peter suggested they rename him. At this moment, Luce is breaking down. He is trying to hold back tears. In a shaking voice he says, "I realized how lucky I am to be an American" and to have the "chance to start over, to redefine myself." When he comes to the words "Here we can be who we choose, here . . . ," he cries. He can't be who he chooses. In crafting the speech, he tries to follow Amy's advice from an earlier scene, where she urges Luce to tell "his own story" (the successful rehabilitation of an adoptee) because this will add a genuine touch to his speech. At the time, Luce is not enthusiastic about it, since he knows that she asks him to say what everyone wants to hear. He just says, "It's good advice." When he tries to follow this advice, he breaks down.

The film does not portray Luce as a helpless victim, though. He manipulates adults in a way that jeopardizes Wilson's career and discredits her accusations of him. He is portrayed as polite but threatening when he brings to Wilson's home flowers from the running team—sending a message that clarifies what this vendetta is about (Deshaun). Even though Wilson shuts the door in his face, he comes in and follows her into her kitchen. She is obviously scared and says, "This is not ok." But Luce insists on talking to her, and they have it out. Even though Wilson seems unconvinced by his words, he makes her listen to what he has to say about tokenism and stereotyping hurting him and other classmates. In a different scene, he is shown as manipulating his adoptive mother. After Amy notices that the fireworks are no longer in the cabinet she put them in, she understands that Luce is lying to her and Peter. At this moment, Luce comes home and finds her sitting next to the cabinet. He asks if she is hiding Christmas presents, since that's where she has always been hiding them—thus he is letting her know how he knew where fireworks were. She says that he acted surprised anyways, and Luce responds that he is good at *acting* surprised. He is making a point about the limits of her power to control his behavior and affect. Luce gives Amy a paper bag that looks like the one with the fireworks, but inside is a container with a fish. "Remember Dennis?" he says invoking the incident with the pet fish he killed, possibly intentionally, possibly accidentally. She chose to trust him then, and he asks her to trust him now: "I thought we could try again. Thanks, Mom." He uses "mom" instead of "Amy," which he has been using since the breach of trust, and by doing so, he signals that he is willing to restore their relationship and be her son if she gets on his side. But he sounds parental and authoritative rather than apologetic at this moment, and the fact that he makes her his co-conspirator makes the viewer wonder again about the balance of power in this relationship and the morality of his actions.

This scene is cut to Luce delivering his graduation speech. The speech is the same one he practiced earlier: he talks about his adoption story. This time, however, he talks about his renaming calmly and changes the words that describe opportunities available to him. He says, "Here we get to be who we are and still be accepted despite our flaws. Here we get to tell our own story. This is mine." However, in this retelling, he withholds his original name from his audience. His speech continues, but the soundtrack's music drowns him out, and we only hear that, at first, he thought his name was "loose"—something detachable. After this—fade to black. The speech, even though it sounds like a success story, has hidden messages that acknowledge Amy's complicity and Luce's alienation. He tells this story without breaking down, perhaps because he abandoned hope of being seen, or perhaps he knows that Amy sees him, even if she cannot understand how he feels, and to him this is enough. The ending is as ambiguous as Luce himself: we are not sure if the film suggests that he is not "loose" any more or that he is just telling the audience what they want to hear, thus minimizing his hybridity. This ambiguity captures the adoptive condition he is living in, and it may be suggesting that he is going to live forever with the way it feels. By having the viewer constantly guess Luce's motives and feelings, the film fosters a recognition of his past, not as static and gone but as present and shaping his relationship with the larger community and its culture that cannot fully accept his hybridity.

The denial of his hybridity is a logical consequence of understanding cultural identity and belonging as rooted in heterocoital human origin and in understanding the transfer of culture as naturally linked to biological, heterocoital origin. This assumed link between nature and culture brackets out hybridity as destabilizing to the symbolic and social order maintained by nurture practices that both draw on and reconstitute the nature-culture link. If the heterocoital genealogy of a child is homogenous culturally and racially, identity and belonging are perceived as a given. If the heterocoital origins of a child suggest a clash of the normative identity and one marked by difference, negotiations of belonging ensue. They may take several forms: erasure of the difference (e.g., passing, complete assimilation), erasure of the normative identity (e.g., one-drop rule, perpetual foreigner), or a permanent code-switching in a situation where no stable cultural category or identity exists (e.g., multiracial, adoptive). All these scenarios are informed by understanding the body as a site of transfer for unhybridized culture. The negotiation of belonging specific to adoptees is unique in that none of the above scenarios creates a heterocoital, biological link of an adoptee to the culture in which they and their families seek belonging. Adoptees' passing would demand an erasure of their heterocoital origin to secure belonging. Keeping the heterocoital origin and racial, cultural, national identifications alive would mark adoptees as not fully belonging in the adoptive culture. Yet, heterocoital origin is culturally perceived as integral to human personhood. Hence the adoption "dance" of building belonging through simultaneous recognition of both adoptive and birth families and cultures, yet with the accompanying need to emotionally divest from the part of identity rooted in heterocoital origin. The cultural demand for erasure or emotional divestment from another set of parents and a pre-adoption past signals the inability of the adoptive culture to accommodate true hybridity—a hybridity that is perceived as a qualitatively new condition, not a collage of identifications and belongings that can be performed selectively in contexts that call for them. Such hybridity blindness stems from a culture's commitment to the nature-culture connection as a guarantee of its survival and uninterrupted futurity; this commitment is manifested as resistance to a reproductive trajectory different from the heterocoital.

Ultimately, the horror genre reinscribes the value of the heterocoital nuclear family as well as the adoptive family that can be an effective imitation of it. The genre that builds its emotional effects—fear and disgust—by engaging with "perceptions of malevolent and antisocial powers" that "emerge from the ill-defined, contradictory lines of the social structure" (Prince 122) is taking up the subject of adoption to scare the viewer with challenges to heterocoital order understood as linking heterocoital reproduction to the transfer of culture. Threats of violence directed at the family and community, incest, or other inappropriate affect and behavior typical of adoption horror plots are informed by "intermediate categories whose anomalies elicit horror and anxiety to the extent that they escape established social classifications" (Prince 122). The insistence on heterocoital family is most noticeable in those plots that involve the adoptee's elimination and the return of the adoptive family to its safe, as-if heterocoital configuration. But the preservation of the adoptive family can also be portrayed as an affirmation of heterocoital order. While adoption horror does portray the adoptive family as a site of affective impotence—incapable of recognizing, disciplining, or rehabilitating the "evil" child through fostering the right kind of affect—the horror adoption plot usually "saves" its viability and cultural value by suggesting that such reproductive failure is the adoptee's "fault," or, more specifically, that their biological origin or pre-adoption past makes them incorrigible. In horror, adoption "does not work," not because the adoptive family fundamentally cannot normalize reproductive difference (and it cannot, since there is no cultural formation that could truly accommodate the adoptee's hybridity) but because the adoptee is a monster that makes a successful imitation of heterocoital family impossible. At the same time, by portraying the adoptee's biological family as an aberration, adoption horror avoids demonizing the heterocoital family as an institution by presenting the malfunctioning biological family as an exception to the rule. In the cases of precarious rehabilitation, the success of the adoptive family is imagined in terms of naturalized parental affect—typically, the adoptive mother's complete devotion to the adoptee—a proof of unconditional love that is assumed essential to the heterocoital parent-child connection.

By playing out the drama of the adoptive family trying and failing to control the adoptee's affect, the horror film disciplines the viewer's affective stances and reactions so they can be aligned with the ethos of the heterocoital order. The portrayals of the adoptees themselves achieve the same goal. Horror film uses the figure of the adoptee to let viewers with known biological origins experience, safely, the threat and terror of the unknown origin. But this exploration is not done for the sake of empathizing with the adoptee; this subjectivity is not the focus, even though it may belong to the main character of the story. The focus is the destructive influence of the adoptee subjectivity and its unpredictable affects. While adoption drama usually resolves its conflict in the formation of the desired adoptee's affective stance—the adopted person's ability to distribute their affective attachment to birth and adoptive family in the way that establishes the primacy of the adoptive family in their own private life and of the heterocoital family in the larger culture—the horror may end by punishing the adoptee who fails to develop such a stance with death or banishment or by putting in question the safety of the adoptive family and community that refuse to take the threat seriously. In horror, the potential of the adoptee's body to reproduce their originary culture, even if it is not activated by nurture, is consistently treated as a crisis, as is a failure of nurture to assure an uninterrupted futurity for the adoptive community. By showing what happens when the origins begin to manifest, horror plays out the conflict that is minimized or resolved in drama through the adoptee's affective divestment from the culture "encoded" in their biology. In this way, adoption horror imagines nurture as weaker than nature in the cultural reproduction process. At the same time, adoption horror draws attention to the absence of social structures that can safely house transracial adoptive hybridity and thus points to the need to reimagine the family space if adoption is to find a home.

•

ART horror films may also be informed by the trope of the child whose nontraditional origin wreaks havoc on their family and community. In such cases, the ART horror film focuses on the terrible ends for the ART-produced child or for their parents (possibly scientists), who pursue reproduction that unsettles the natural state of the things by changing human biology and breaking social taboos. While the adoption horror film is envisioning nature as a Russian roulette—you never know what you are going to get—ART horror is anxious about getting something unpredicted and unpredictable while aiming for a specific, scientifically possible outcome. Both are showing the failure of nurture to socialize the nontraditionally reproduced or kinned person because the nontraditional origin, or horrible heredity with unknown and unpredictable consequences, exceeds the power of culture to translate reproductive difference into the heterocoital framework. Like the threatening adoptee of the horror genre, the entity reproduced through ART destroys families and social order when introduced into the human social space, but ART horror films are often concerned with containment of the "product of the experiment" in the lab, rather than within a human family structure. Even though a great deal of socialization attempted by parent-scientists follows the scripts typical of a nuclear family's, the blurred boundaries between home and lab spaces in ART horror films allow us to see more clearly the discursive work around biology that naturalizes heterocoital origin and kinship scripts. ART horror films, perhaps more directly than those dealing with adoption, reveal anxieties about threats to the patriarchal heterocoital framework posed by reproductive technologies that may lead to transgressions of heteronormativity, incest taboo, monogamy, and social taboos against trans identities. At the same time, this subgenre is working through its own unique obsessions and anxieties brought on by technologically assisted, non-heterocoital reproduction.

The 1976 horror B movie *Embryo*, for example, is concerned about the social impact of a nontraditionally gestated human. The sequence of horrific events that earned this film its attribution to the horror genre follows the discovery of her own reproductive difference and disability by Victoria (Barbara Carrera), a young woman whose mother committed suicide while pregnant with Victoria. Victoria, while still an embryo too young to be saved by conventional medical procedures, is illegally transferred to the private home lab of Dr. Paul Holliston (Rock Hudson) to be gestated in a high-tech tank that functions as an artificial womb. Paul has successfully gestated a dog embryo this way, aided by an experimental growth hormone that speeds up the process. He is working on biotechnology that might help keep premature babies alive and even take miscarriages to full term. While the dog experiment is successful, Victoria's has an unexpected glitch: she continues to grow at an alarming rate even after she is removed from the tank. Within a few days she reaches the age of about twenty-two years. Paul finds a way to stop this rapid aging (he uses a strong, dangerous drug), but he must deal with the problem of socializing a twenty-two-year-old who has not gone through childhood. He manages to do this while keeping his experiment secret, which requires isolation from his family. He sends away Martha (Diane Ladd), his late wife's sister, who lives with him, and minimizes contact with his son and daughter-in-law, who are expecting a baby. For a while, everything goes well, and Victoria is adjusting fast. She befriends the dog, a black Doberman (evocative of Damien's black dog guardian from *The Omen*). She can even pass as Paul's new research assistant, and as such takes part in social events and meets his family. One of the unintended results of hers and the dog's experiment is their unusually high level of intelligence, and Victoria soon begins to understand her condition (rapid aging) and the consequences of her reproductive difference. From conversations with Paul and from reading his notes, she concludes that she can be locked up in a lab and experimented on if anyone finds out what she is. So, with Paul's help, she successfully conceals her difference until she gets pregnant (by Paul), and the presence of elevated growth hormone levels triggers her rapid aging again.

It is telling that the horror sequence in the film is initiated at the moment when the nontraditionally reproduced human becomes capable of reproduction herself. Within the plot logic, however, the revelation of her pregnancy does not happen until the very end. First, Victoria experiences stabbing pain in her stomach and tries to alleviate it with the same drug Paul used to stop her aging. Eventually, though, the drug stops helping, and she uses the power of the largest computer in the country to search for a possible remedy, which turns out to be a substance that needs to be extracted from the pituitary gland of a human embryo. Initially, she tries to act in the most "ethical" way she can imagine and obtain the extract from a pregnant prostitute's embryo that is already dead in the womb. She fails, and the woman herself dies. Desperate, Victoria decides to use the embryo of Paul's daughter-in-law, Helen (Anne Schedeen), who comes to check on Victoria just as she is dealing with the aftermath of her failed attempt to obtain the remedy. By this moment, Paul knows what Victoria is up to. He alerts his son, Gordon (John Elerick), and rushes home, but they are too late. Victoria, who has already aged significantly, has removed Helen's embryo and put it in the gestation tank. As the men are trying to subdue her, she stabs Gordon with a syringe, breaks the tank, and drives away. Paul finally catches up with her and crashes her car. At this point, Victoria is dying of old age, but she demonstrates a surprising will to live and manages to crawl away from the burning car toward a pond. Paul chases her and attempts to drown her until he is pulled away by the police, yelling, "She's got to die! You don't understand!" Meanwhile, the EMTs discover that the senescent woman is writhing on the ground because "she is having a baby!" The camera focuses on Victoria's hand clutching Paul's, and Paul's contorted face as he is crying, "It can't happen! Die! Goddamn you, die! Both of you!" At this moment, she is telling him that it is his baby, and his jaw drops. Victoria is taken away on a stretcher to the sound of his anguished "Nooo!"

For all its campiness, this scene suggests some moral dilemmas prompted by the "intrusion" of technology into the natural reproductive process. It makes sense of Victoria's dogged persistence in looking for a remedy to her condition: a mother would do anything for her child. But it also shows her struggling to make a choice between saving herself and letting her child die versus harming other people to extract a remedy. Rather than suggesting a clear moral decision, the film opts for portraying the moral confusion caused by the "brave new world" situation. At the sight of Paul and Gordon rushing into the lab, she cries out, "I don't want to kill! I don't want to kill! I don't want to live!"—a realization that she has gone too far and does not see a clear way out. Her motherhood is presented as monstrous, and she is a monster not only because she is killing but also because her pregnancy is horrifically unnatural. An old, dying woman giving birth to a child that grew from embryo to term within several days is a scientific breakthrough that hardly looks appealing to the audience and is condemned by the very scientist who has dared to disturb the natural order of things. The ultimate terror is not her, though. The ending of the film is a fade-to-black frame with the sound of a baby's bottom slapped followed by the infant crying. This unseen baby, her progeny, is a sign of an uncertain, unpredictable future. While Victoria's motivation for violence could be understood as a mother's desire to save her child, the open-ended life of that child is a blank slate that the viewer can fill with an array of their own anxieties about nontraditional reproduction.

The idea that technologically mediated reproduction is monstrous also informs a more recent film, *Splice* (2009), that further develops anxieties about scientific interventions into nature-given biology. *Splice* is a story of an artificially reproduced chimera—a human-animal hybrid, Dren (Delphine Chanéac). Dren is a product of an experiment run by researchers Clive Nicoli (Adrien Brody) and Elsa Kast (Sarah Polley), who are coworkers and a couple. The focus of their research is production of artificial biological organisms that can be used as sources of proteins in the production of pharmaceuticals. Elsa, the more ambitious and less ethically minded of the two, goes rogue and creates an embryo of an organism by mixing synthetic animal cells with her own. The result is a creature that has human and animal qualities: it is intelligent but cannot easily speak; it has an expressive human-like face, bird-like legs, and an animal-like tail; it behaves sometimes as a human child and sometimes as a feral animal. Even though Clive tries to maintain the scientific perspective and stop Elsa from continuing the experiment, she manipulates and pushes him to comply with her vision (which draws criticism from Clive's brother, who considers Clive weak). Eventually, Dren is seen by the couple and the viewers as Clive and Elsa's child. Scenes abound that show them caring for her as if she were a human. Yet, at the same time, the film continues to emphasize that we are dealing with something unpredictable. When Dren gets sick, the couple submerge her in water to cool her down—a gesture of care. But Clive holds Dren down to drown her, taking the chance to course-correct what Elsa has started. Dren dies and then comes back to life, having unexpectedly developed a set of gills to survive the drowning. Anxieties over the technological method of reproduction are channeled through such transformations of Dren. As she grows up, and typically in response to stressful situations, she sprouts wings and eventually even changes her sex to male. *Splice* blatantly imagines nontraditional reproduction as a slippery slope that leads to a production of a monster, horrific in its hybridity and ultimately an uncontrollable threat to human life. No less horrific is the treatment of Dren by her human parent-scientists who, while they genuinely care for her, still think of her as an experimental subject, a source of valuable proteins, and a property of the lab. The execution of heterocoital family scripts inflected with the relationships between scientists and the object of their experimentation suggests that nontraditionally reproduced entities are not accepted within the heterocoital framework as fully human.

At the end of *Splice,* Dren dies and resurrects yet again, this time transformed into a male. Having been humiliated by her unsuccessful seduction of Clive and punitive maiming by Elsa, who cuts off the poisonous tip of Dren's tail, the male Dren, capable of more aggressive actions, rapes Elsa and kills Clive. The return of the monster unsettles both the heterocoital order, by transgressing multiple taboos through Dren's performance of a horrific heterocoital act, and the order of scientific experimentation, by bringing its effects into the world with unbridled chaos of violence. Elsa kills Dren, but the banishment of the monster is not complete. The ending scene of the film shows Elsa in the office of the head of the corporation she has been working for, signing the agreement to carry to term the baby conceived during her rape. The last frame is the camera's zoom out on two silhouettes outlined against a window with a gloomy cityscape beyond: pregnant Elsa and, behind her, the head of the corporation, Joan Chorot (Simona Maicanescu), positioned as an unlikely couple in an iconic hetero image: Joan's hands are on Elsa's shoulders, and they are staring into the uncertain and dangerous but scientifically irresistible future. Like *Embryo, Splice* ends on a note of impending danger that may come from the uncertain progeny, signaling the risk of interfering with the natural biological order of things. And even though *Splice* is more convincing in performing its gesture of exclusion—Dren is a more obvious monster than human-looking and human-feeling Victoria in *Embryo*—the narrative logic takes both of them to the same end. In both, the likelihood of integrating ART-produced individuals into human social realm as persons is low.

The "return" to reproduction as a heterocoital act in both films, albeit the one tainted and revised by technoreproduction, is managing the fear of the heterocoital order breakdown. In *Embryo,* the child of Victoria and Paul is conceived through consensual sex that Victoria asks for to "learn" about this sphere of human relationships. Yet, the viewer's awareness that she has been gestated and raised by him gives this heterocoital act a transgressive feel. In *Splice,* the rape scene is evocative of transphobic anxieties over revisions to heterocoital reproduction. Beyond the shock of Dren's sex change and their having had sex with both Clive and Elsa, the most fraught moment comes when, on top of Elsa, Dren speaks for the first time and says, "I want to be inside of you." This statement is an establishing of dominance by a male over a female, a declaration of Dren's, now male, sex drive, and at the same time it is a complex demand to enter the heterocoital order. Dren is claiming such entrance as a man who can reproduce through a heterocoital act with a woman, but he may also be channeling the desire to have been a child gestated by a mother, not in an artificial womb in a lab. By raping Elsa and leaving her with a baby, he establishes his right to have progeny reproduced the human way. Such bizarre hybridity (and let's not forget that Dren has Elsa's own genetic material) may be indicative of the scientific ethical concerns over germ-line genetic modifications that can be transferred through generations of progeny with unpredictable results. Dren's progeny is a black box. But it is also channeling a patriarchal anxiety of being displaced by an unpredictable outcome of scientific research that destroys the rules of engagement set by the heterocoital framework.

The conservatism of ART horror films is expressed in rehashing the patriarchy's fears of disempowerment by engaging the scenario in which a scientist who is "playing God" is punished by their scientific discovery. In *Embryo* and *Splice,* the child is the punishment and demise of Paul and Clive but also of what Evelyn Blackwood calls "the Patriarchal Man."[16] While Paul's predicament in *Embryo* is the corruption of his progeny and future, and Clive in

16. An abstracted man-figure that constellates rules and characteristics of patriarchy and begins to exist as a structuring point of reference in relation to which all social phenomena are understood.

Splice gets killed, it is interesting to notice that they both suffer at the hands of women who would not stop at the ethical line in experimentation. *Splice,* too, follows a patriarchal scenario with the dangerous ambitious feminine in charge of non-heterocoital reproduction as a source of chaos. It goes further than *Embryo,* which still features heterocoital reproduction, by suggesting that a woman may exclude the man from reproduction and reproduce herself as a monster. Clive, who is literally accused by his brother of being emasculated by Elsa, is portrayed as a weak representative of the Patriarchal Man, caving to Elsa's wishes and unable to reestablish the ethical parameters of the experiment (which would preserve the heterocoital order). Victoria is also an example of a woman trying to use reproductive science to dangerous ends. Both Elsa and Victoria suggest a dangerous revision to the patriarchal order, where women's access to science bodes ill for the future of the humanity. In such scenarios, men are concerned with reestablishing the rules, and the woman, who transgresses without regret, is the source of disaster. Paul in *Embryo* tries to stop Victoria from cutting his son's baby from his daughter-in-law's womb and from surviving to give birth to their baby. Clive in *Splice* is the consistent voice of reason who is trying to tame his partner Elsa's drive to push experimentation past morally acceptable boundaries. The men are thus reestablishing what Lacan termed the "law of the Father," which is commonly conflated with nature, while the "unnatural" woman scientist is trying to break the order with disastrous results. When Dren becomes the heterocoital father, the whole order is perverted, and this monstrous reproduction represents a persistent concern of ART horror films: a displacement of the father at conception that is understood as men's loss of control over reproduction. Art horror films work out this fear through turning the empowered feminine, in control of her own reproduction, into a monster.

The ending of *False Positive,* a 2021 film about IVF, seems less conservative, as it seems to celebrate a woman wresting power over her reproduction away from her husband and the crazed doctor-scientist, both of whom are portrayed as paternalistic, condescending men not ready to outgrow patriarchal narcissism, which seeks control over the woman and sees her as a function rather than a subject. Lucy (Llana Glazer), a copy writer, and her husband, Adrian (Justin Theroux), a surgeon, reach out to Adrian's mentor, renowned fertility specialist Dr. John Hindle (Pierce Brosnan), who has developed his own ART technique, which produces consistent results. Hindle performs the procedure on Lucy. The pregnancy takes, but soon the couple faces another problem: overstimulation caused three embryos to attach, and the couple need to choose which one is going to be carried to term. The choice is between twin boys and a girl. Lucy wants to keep the girl, but Adrian is trying to convince her to keep the boys. Eventually, Adrian acquiesces. Hindle performs "selective reduction" that is supposed to stop the development of the male embryos, but, since the procedure, Lucy has begun to suspect that something is wrong. In due time, she gives birth to twin boys, which confirms her suspicion that Adrian conspired with Hindle to reduce the girl embryo. Not only that, but Hindle inseminated Lucy with his own genetic material. He has been using his own sperm to inseminate female patients, and he controls the process to increase the number of male births because he wants to spread his bloodline across the world. Horrified, Lucy confronts Hindle at the clinic, kicks him in the groin, pushes him into the gynecological chair, and beats him up; she also destroys his sperm storage. She finds the reduced girl embryo in a biospecimen bag in Hindle's lab and takes it home. The final scene is her nursing the embryo, which appears to suckle on her breast.

While the film has a monster figure that needs to be discovered and destroyed—Dr. Hindle—the source of persistent horror in *False Positive* is more diffuse. It is the effects of the patriarchy itself, impersonated by not only the megalomaniacal male doctor hell-bent on spreading "superior" male genes but also several other characters: the husband, who becomes the doctor's ally in reinforcing patriarchal values; Lucy's male coworkers, who subject Lucy to paternalistic insults under the guise of feminist wokeness; and a number of women who are brainwashed by patriarchy, to different degrees but enough to help Hindle and Adrian control Lucy. By presenting Lucy as alone and isolated in her struggles with the whole patriarchal apparatus as she is trying to have a baby girl, *False Positive* is stirring up anxieties about ARTs from a somewhat different perspective than *Embryo* and *Splice*. While the motif of the arrogant scientist is still present, this time the scientist is not an agent of chaos but a deliberate creator of a reproductive order that reduces women to wombs without brains and values their lives less than males'. The horror here is the vulnerability of the maternal body that lost control over the reproductive power at the level of biology. When biology is controlled and revised by science, women, who are kept in the dark, may not have a say in the social and political effects of such reproduction.

Through the recurrent anchoring scene of Lucy on the examination table in Dr. Hindle's office, the film incrementally builds a feeling of despair at Lucy's gradual loss of power over her reproductive process, her body, and herself. The first visit to a clinic is set to a blissful soundtrack. Lucy's every desire is met. She is greeted and examined by female nurses in pink, feminine uniforms that look like sexy yet tasteful old-timey nurse costumes. In the initial examination scene, the camera is trained on Lucy's face pried and prodded by devices that take her vitals. Her face is glowing with serene, happy anticipation. Hindle is charming, if in a narcissistic way, during their first meeting. "I will give you the best possible chance of getting pregnant," he reassures Lucy. A little creepiness develops during Lucy's pelvic exam, however. She is lying down with Adrian by her side holding her hand. Nurse Dawn (Gretchen Mol) squirts lubricant over the speculum in Hindle's hands. They smile at each other, and Hindle grunts approvingly. He proceeds to spread the lubricant on the speculum with two fingers (for a long time!) with a satisfied smile on his face. Adrian is trying to look away but eventually turns his head surprised that the spreading of the lubricant takes a while. He stares at Hindle's fingers, and there is a hint of puzzlement on his face, but he quickly turns away and then looks at Lucy. Overall, Adrian looks uncertain about what he should be doing during the whole procedure or what his role is in this interaction between Hindle and Lucy. As Hindle inserts the speculum, Lucy's face shows mild discomfort, and Adrien is staring away into a corner, uncomfortable with the situation.

To put him at ease, Hindle begins telling a story about the time he and Adrian still worked together that showcases Adrian's good character and ability to do the right thing even if it goes against institutionalized rules (Adrian conducted a reconstruction mastectomy on a patient against the hospital's orders). The story, however, evolves into Hindle complaining that in his work he often "wish[es he] could clone [him]self." "That's the only way I can get the job done," he says. It may seem like an innocuous narcissistic gesture on his part—Hindle makes it, as he does everything, about himself—but in this particular case, the shifting of the story's focus away from Adrian is a foreshadowing of his displacement of Adrian as the biological father of Lucy's baby. He will, during their next encounter, secretly fertilize Lucy with his own sperm instead of Adrian's. This first examination scene also foreshadows another source of horror in the film—the blatantly paternalistic treatment Lucy is going to suffer from all male characters in the film. At the end of the exam, Hindle inappropriately slaps Lucy on the knee to let her know they are finished. He dismisses her concerns over the seeming ease of the ART process he offers, given that she has been diagnosed with infertility by many doctors, and touts his own greatness as a fertility doctor while showing her photos of all the happy women he helped get pregnant. He explains his unique method as part IUI and part IVF and calls it, unabashedly, "in-utero Hindle fertilization," which, to someone who is rewatching the film, spells loud and clear what he is doing.

Later, the fertilization scene heightens the feeling that something is not right. Adrian begins to show cracks in his "good man" facade. He receives a jar for his sperm specimen from a nurse who seems ready to assist him personally in the process of sperm retrieval. And, while he dismisses the nurse and thus confirms his "faithful husband" image, he extracts his sample to a video of a woman being choked and slapped. The woman in the video is pushed onto the couch under the camera along a trajectory similar to the one in which Lucy is lowered onto the examination table in the next shot, except the hands handling Lucy appear to be gentle. The link between this gentleness and the violence of the preceding shot lingers and creates an uncertainty in the viewer, who cannot yet believe what they have seen. Hindle asks Lucy if she wants to watch and aims a big mirror at her vagina. He leaves the mirror in place, even though Lucy says no, and goes through the same manipulations with the speculum, making eyes at Adrian who seems to have become more comfortable with watching Hindle stroke the instrument. Holding a syringe of sperm, Hindle praises Adrian: "Good work, son!" He adds, "This is powerful stuff," which seems to make little sense: How would he know if Adrian's "stuff" is powerful before the results of the procedure are known? But this mindless sperm worship is really Hindle's brag about the potency of his own genetic material. The sperm transfer sequence is a series of close-ups and intercuts between Lucy's and Hindle's faces, suggestive of something more than a sperm injection. Hindle is obviously having an emotional experience that culminates in a soft grunt as if he himself ejaculated.

The shifting stances of Hindle and Adrian in relation to Lucy add to the growing tension as Lucy develops suspicions that Adrian may not be her ally. When Hindle announces that Lucy is pregnant, Adrian's impulse is to hug Hindle first, then he kisses Lucy, which foreshadows Adrian's betrayal. The rift between Lucy and Adrian becomes pronounced when they discuss which embryos should be carried to term. The first ultrasound reveals three embryos—"twin boys" and a "female singlet," in Hindle's words. The male embryos are immediately humanized and personified—a manipulation to make Lucy think of them as more viable and desirable. Hindle enhances the manipulation by explaining that "selective reduction" is needed to avoid preemies or miscarriages. He calls it a "sacrifice to ensure a successful birth" and immediately recommends keeping the boys, who "look healthy," while the girl "is a bit small." Lucy is hesitating and is obviously distressed not only at the need to make a choice but also at the realization that the promised pregnancy is more than she expected, and it looks rather like a burden now. Hindle reassures her but then asks Adrian to "have a word" outside of the examination room—the first inkling of conspiracy they will develop to trick Lucy into carrying boys to term. The next scene is the couple's celebratory dinner. Lucy, still trying to come to terms with the situation, says, "I am pregnant," and Adrian responds, "Yes, we are pregnant." What might sound like a gesture of solidarity (Lucy is not in it on her own) in this specific context begins to sound like an ownership claim—Adrian claims his right to make decisions about Lucy's body because the children inside it are also his. While Lucy is still processing the decision they must make, Adrian says that he "agree[s] with Dr. Hindle," and they should keep the boys. Lucy wants to keep the girl and shares her fantasy of lying in bed with her daughter, who has "clear eyes" that can see "right past [her] to some better version of [her]self." To her, the daughter, whom she wants to name Wendy after a character from *Peter Pan,* is a promise of a better future.

This scene is connected to the next one with an intercut of a strange, receding shot of Adrian typing away at his computer in total darkness, glancing over his shoulder as if afraid of being caught. The shot reinforces a sense of conspiracy, which is revealed later as the conspiracy between Adrian and Hindle, husband and doctor, to make Lucy give birth to the boys. The significance of this single act is, however, greater. They are also planning to open a joint practice and scale up Hindle's project of populating the world with his progeny. In this way, the film is negotiating the potential loss of power of individual men to claim their progeny based on the biogenetic link—the bedrock of the patriarchal heterocoital order. Adrian cedes his place as a heterocoital father to reach for a more abstract version of reproductive power as a fertility specialist. His personal power and prowess are transfigured as the power of patriarchal technological reproduction.

The selective embryo reduction scene is cast in dark tones, in contrast to other scenes in the doctor's office. The way the men are positioned around the examination table reinforces the coming together of two men as appropriators of Lucy's body. Adrian is no longer between Hindle and Lucy; he is at the foot of the table with Hindle, that is, he is "on Hindle's side," and Lucy is in the dark about their joint intentions. In a later, yet another examination room scene, this configuration will change to suggest a further erosion of Lucy's ownership of her reproductive power. In this one, the camera is at the foot of the table trained on Lucy's fully supine body. Her head cannot be seen. We see her legs and belly, and, instead of her upper body, Adrian's torso and head occupy the top of the shot. Adrian looks like a chimera (see figure 2.2), the top half of the body is his and the bottom half is Lucy's—an image suggestive of his encroaching appropriation of Lucy's body and reproductivity. Hindle is on the side, examining Lucy. At the end of the scene, Hindle and Adrian lock in a long hug that obviously excludes Lucy, who is taken aback by this borderline inappropriate display of male bonding. Her suspicions bubble to the surface in a dream sequence, a sort of premonition she has, that features her following Adrian to a hotel, where he is given a key and a room number by one of

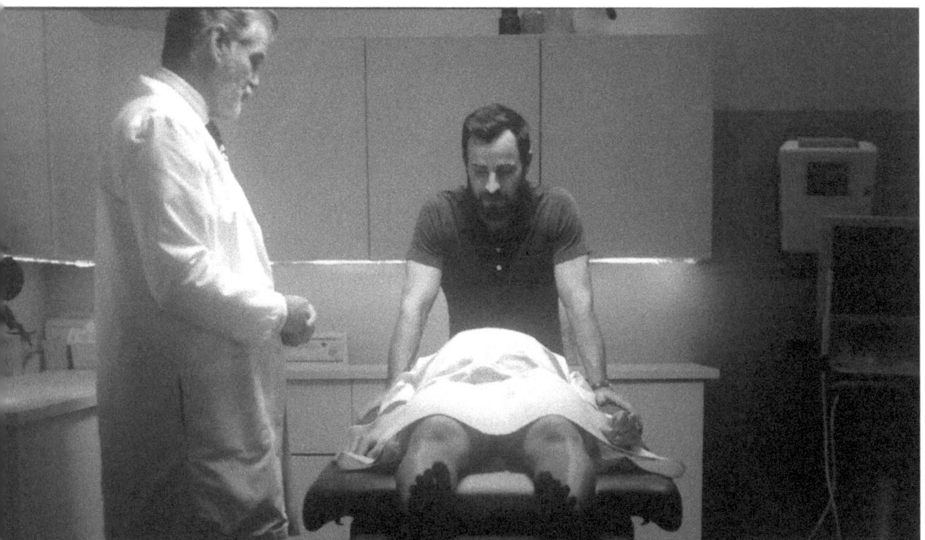

IGURE 2.2. Adrian as a chimera in *False Positive.* A24, 2021.

Hindle's nurses. The nurse kisses Adrian on the lips as she sends him on his way. Through a peephole, Lucy observes Adrian fellating Hindle in the hotel room until they both notice her, but they do not act embarrassed, just stare at her disapprovingly. The representation of the husband and doctor's collusion to appropriate Lucy's reproductive labor as a sexual encounter between two men suggests that it is necessary to "bond" participants in child conception through acts of sex, even if they are not heterocoital or even real. Sexual conception is still looming large as a necessary ingredient to define men's role in the process, even though the extent of Adrian's and Hindle's engagement is the technical and business side of things. To transfer his heterocoital reproductive power, Adrian has to submit to Hindle, the über-man with better genes. Hindle is also the "Father"-mentor whose ideas and rules Adrian has to accept as his own in order to ride the coattails of his patriarchal power. Adrian's sexual submission to Hindle reestablishes "by proxy" his place in the imagined-as-heterocoital act of conceiving children to which Adrian will be a social father.

Such negotiation of changes in male reproductive power is represented as terrifying in *False Positive.* This potential response to the cultural fear of men losing control over reproduction creates another kind of horror—that of a woman becoming a womb at the hands of men who deliberately take away her subjectivity, autonomy, and freedom under the guise of care and desire to help her fulfil her reproductive desires. The buildup of patriarchal oppression in *False Positive* is ultimately resolved via a revenge climax as Lucy destroys Hindle's lab, his sperm storage, and, likely, his testicles. She beats him bloody in the gynecological chair and leaves, covered in blood, with the embryo of her unborn daughter and the paperwork that establishes Adrian and Hindle's joint practice. At home, she stands up to her husband's manipulation of her. Adrian's plan to coerce her into delivering the boys hinges on the assumption that once the babies are there, her maternal instinct will take over or her maternal conscience will not see abandoning them as a choice. Lucy rejects this coercive patriarchal vision of her "maternal nature" by rejecting the male children. First, it happens in a *Peter Pan*–inspired dream sequence: she releases the boys out of the window, turning them into "the lost boys" who float away over nighttime Manhattan. But in a later, more realistic scene, she hands over the twin boys to Adrian and tells him to get out. She rejects her role as reproducer of male bodies and patriarchal subjectivities as well as the assumed duty of maternal care for Adrian's, or, rather, Hindle's, progeny. To his weak "But what am I supposed to do?" she yells, "Go!"

The film's persistent allusion to *Peter Pan* suggests Adrian's resemblance to Peter, a character who benefits from support and "mothering" of feminine figures in his life yet fails to recognize and acknowledge their care; worse yet, he considers the effects of such care his own achievement. By handing the twins over to him, Lucy forces Adrian to realize the scope of labor required for reproduction. This is her rejection of the role of Wendy, a girl Peter lures to join him, who is represented as an "indispensable housewife" (Chassagnol 207), an epitome of the patriarchal woman, similar to the pre-transformation Lucy, who even chose to name her daughter Wendy in honor of this character from *Peter Pan*. Through this gesture, Lucy rejects a Wendy-like future for her daughter as well. The ending, in which Lucy is nursing her unborn daughter, suggests the perpetuation of the feminine and her reproductive choice to sustain female life. However, the nursing of the embryo is a dream sequence, a hallucination, so the likelihood of a feminine-empowered future remains uncertain. The ending (weakly) asserts Lucy's control over her reproduction and body, but the film stops short of offering a vision of empowered, yet not monstrous, femininity. Like adoption horror plots that aim to rehabilitate and incorporate the adoptee, who remains an ever-present spring of uncertainty and a constant possibility of the heterocoital order demise, ART horror films tend to end on an anxious note.

While both adoption and ART horror cinema concern themselves with threats to the heterocoital reproductive order, they focus on divergent aspects. Adoption horror films present as failed attempts to socialize into the heterocoital culture a child whose origins and kinship do not coincide with the expected heterocoital configurations. Beyond the anxieties of adoption horror cinema, ART horror films present nontraditional reproduction as a threat to the whole paradigm of heteropatriarchy, beyond just being a threat to the biological nuclear family. They make more visible the gender-inflected struggle over the new ways to conceptualize reproductive power. Specifically, the ART horror film is working out the ways to deal with the absence or substitution of the man-Father at conception. It suggests that by displacing heterocoitus as a point of origin, reproductive technologies put "the law of the Father" in question and generate uncertainty at the point when the control of female reproductive power by the patriarchy begins to falter. In other words, the question becomes whether the role of the woman in the new reproductive process can stay under the patriarchy's control. The increase of the woman's power is often imagined as a consequence of a man's losing control over his sperm, which can then be used by anyone the way they see fit. The anxiety of the man's loss of control over his genetic material is often represented as his displacement at conception, which can take the form of unsanctioned sperm use (*Embryo*), its substitution for another man's genetic material (*False Positive*), or even a total lack of need for it (*Splice*). The next chapter will show that in the comedy genre, typically less conservative than the horror genre, the difference between representations of adoption and ART reproduction falls along similar lines. And while adoption comedy manages to present some nonpatriarchal possibilities for nontraditional kinship even as it ridicules them, ART comedy's thrust is to brainstorm ways for the Patriarchal Man to keep control over the outcomes of nontraditional reproduction even if kinship configurations are revised.

CHAPTER 3

Adoption and ARTs in Comedy

Testing the Limits of the Heterocoital Order

Huh? My story? Okay. It was never easy
for me. I was born a poor Black child.
—Steve Martin as Navin Johnson in *The Jerk*

I'm gonna be a mama too.
—Arnold Schwarzenegger as Dr. Alex Hesse in *Junior*

"I was born a poor Black child," claims Navin—the protagonist of adoption comedy *The Jerk* (1979)—while telling his life story, but Navin is a white man who was adopted by a family of Black sharecroppers in Mississippi. Adoption comedy thrives on such confusion about one's origin and on "inversio[n] of narrative structures" (Mamber 80) familiar to the viewer. In *The Jerk,* the recognizable trope of a white middle-class family adopting a less privileged child of a different race is reversed, and the white middle-class adoptive family is displaced from the savior-adopter position by a Black family of modest means. This reversal generates events that expose and put in question cultural assumptions about the link between heterocoital genealogy and one's position in social hierarchy, which is considered a result of culture transfer along kinship lines.

Comedy as a genre is notoriously hard to define, and it is often spoken of as a "mode" (King 2), which can be present in other genres, or as a "way of looking at the universe" (Horton and Rapf 2). Like horror and (melo)drama, comedy is often defined not only by structural features but by "the emotional reaction it is intended to provoke" (King 2). Comparing horror and comedy, Geoff King writes that both may depend on a typical Hollywood structure that "revolve[s] around the creation followed by the resolution of a specific emotional tension" (8), but while the emotional landscape created by horror is more punishing for the viewer, the comedy opens up a space where the emotional tension is discharged in a pleasurable way. Like horror, comedy is concerned with adoption as a phenomenon with a larger social effect, and they both "differ from tragedies in their emphasis on the social rather than on the individual" (Horton and Rapf 3). While both comedic and horrific emotional effects originate in a tension about a transgression of social order, comedy invites the viewer to engage with it not through fear and disgust but through laughter and play—"a larger step back from potential seriousness, tension and anxiety" (King 8). For example, while adoption horror thrives on anxiety created by the unknown, invisible origin of the adoptee, comedy makes this origin obvious and incongruent with its context. The visibility of its incongruency becomes the butt of the joke. For instance, the inability of the adoptive family to integrate itself and the adoptee into the adoptive culture, which is perceived as a tragedy in drama and a threat in horror, is exposed in comedy as a ludicrous task. Its impossibility emphasizes the ridiculously high cultural standards for good parenting, while both adoptive and birth parents are presented as coping the best way they can with cultural expectations, often failing. The comedic effect may also be a result of a mismatch between culturally expected and performed affect, or of parody that draws on cultural stereotypes.

Adoption comedy conflicts typically disrupt expected scripts for race, class, gender, and sexuality based on the assumption of biocultural origin consistency that naturalizes the link between these categories and heterocoital reproduction. The focus of such disruptions is the figure of the adoptee who is "mis"-placed with a family whose biology, social status, and culture bring into high relief the adoptee's difference; the humor is often produced around the attempts to bridge such difference. In turn, the ART comedies analyzed in this chapter are built around disruptions to expected heterocoital connections of men to their children, and they go a bit further than adoption comedies in revealing the stakes of the patriarchy's insistence on imagining families as heterocoital even if they are "as-if." ART comedies show the patriarchy's possible responses to non-heterocoital revisions of human reproduction and kinship, including a shift toward imagining reproduction without women. While adoption comedies ultimately land on the side of the status quo, their exploration of unconventional and playful modes of existence leaves in its wake a pool of possibilities for alternative ways of being. By making them available to the viewer through, however short, pleasurable emotional engagement with the alternatives to heterocoital scripts, adoption comedy sets the stage for possible liberatory revisions of heterocoital imaginary. The analysis of *Delivery Man* and *Junior* later in the chapter shows that ART comedies do open similar possibilities for reinventing heterocoital frameworks, but they tend to look at them with greater apprehension. The ART comedies discussed here introduce more sinister visions of revised patriarchy, even as they show sentimentalized transformations of traditional patriarchal fatherhood. While adoption comedies' conservative endings may still continue to evoke hopeful alternatives to the heterocoital, patriarchal reality, albeit presented as ridiculous and marginalized, ART comedies' resolutions to the complications introduced by non-heterocoital reproduction reveal the ways in which the patriarchy can be strengthened, even to the point of erasure of whatever power women have due to their role in the heterocoital reproductive process. The progression of this chapter through a discussion of adoption comedy followed by the turn toward comedic representations of assisted reproduction suggests a shift in the ideological focus between these two subgenres of nontraditional reproduction comedy: from preserving the heterocoital family as it exists toward revising it and enhancing the power of the patriarchy by changing the role of men in reproduction.

As a subgenre, adoption comedy comes the closest, perhaps, to romantic comedy, with a plot built around some typical "mistaken identity" devices, including "characters donning disguises or swapping identities," "crossed conversations," and misrecognitions (Weitz 73). While adoption comedies feature a great deal of slapstick and farce, the prevailing ethos aligns with the way Celestino Deleyto defines romantic comedy: as "less a narrative of the heterosexual couple with a happy ending than a particular type of story about interpersonal affective and erotic relationships" (176). In adoption comedy, which works out challenges to heterosexuality in nontraditional reproduction, heterosexual couplings are ubiquitous and still drive the plot, but they are framed by the heterocoital versus nonnormative kinship conflicts and are surrounded by nonnormative expressions of sexual and reproductive desires. The desirability and inevitability of heterocoital order is built up as adoption comedy rolls through a series of narrative events featuring nonreproductive or otherwise queered[1] affective attachments and erotic orientations.

The comedic effect is also often achieved by challenging cultural expectations for someone's social performance of an expected cultural script that would signal their belonging in a family and community. For example, an adoptee may seem out of place because their social performances are at odds with cultural expectations for the kind of bodies they have. Or adoption comedy scenarios may create plot-driving conflicts by inverting vectors of power

1. I use the term *queer* in the sense of it Shelley Park has introduced into critical adoption studies: as describing practices of intimacy and kinning that resist "narratives that Michael Warner (1991)" names "'reprosexuality' and 'repronarrativity'" (24) and open space for imagining kinship that exceeds heterocoital scripts.

that determine who can adopt whom and who is allowed to perform or claim as their own a certain culture. Because adoptive family is culturally imagined as an imitation of the heterocoital family, its configuration depends on which heterocoital unions are socially acceptable. Cases in which a mismatch between parents and children is apparent tell us who has the power to rescue and own children. Such inversions often happen along the lines of race, class, gender, and (when transnational adoption is involved) citizenship. Through plot inversions that introduce scenarios of unconventional kinship, adoption comedy, like no other genre, manifests what the often unexamined concept of "culture" means, what is exactly reproduced and transferred through the institution of heterocoital nuclear family, and what is at stake in maintaining this kind of family as the norm. Adoption comedy shows that "culture" transmitted via heterocoital kinship means naturalization (and assumed hereditary transmission) of categories that can be socially constructed.

The endings of adoption comedy typically domesticate nonconventional family-making by affirming adoptive kinship, but this validation is given on condition that the adoptive family lives by heterocoital cultural norms. An adoptive family reunion and a restrengthening of the adoptive tie often happens through the mechanism characteristic of adoption narratives: origin discovery with subsequent emotional divestment from the adoptee's biological family, culture, or both. Heterosexual marriage or a romantic heterosexual coupling of an adoptee may become a guarantee of heterocoital futurity, which brackets out adoption as a genealogical exception, as in most of the films discussed in this chapter. The integration of the adoptee's "nature" into the adoptive family may be presented as minimization of the importance of origin, combined with a "renaturing" of the adoptee—in other words, a reimagining of the adoptee's acquired traits as genetically transmitted in order to boost their resemblance to the adoptive family. For example, in *The Jerk* and *Flirting with Disaster* (Russell 1996), upon the return of the adoptees from the search for "who they really are," the traits that emphasize the white adoptees' Blackness or Jewishness are imagined not as just social performance but as genetically conditioned behavior that is a testimony to their naturalized belonging with the adoptive family. If transnational or transracial adoption is involved, the adoptee's origin and anxiety about possible nonbelonging may be externalized and displaced onto a character who is a foreigner (*Fakin' da Funk* [1997] and *Catfish in Black Bean Sauce* [1999]). Alternatively, the restoration of the heterocoital family may be straightforward, like in *Raising Arizona* (1987). More often than not, however, adoption comedy endings celebrate non-heterocoital families and present them as socially valuable forms of kinship, but such nonnormative kinship is still imagined through heterocoital metaphors.

In trying to understand how adoption comedy operates, it is also worth remembering that humor-induced laughter is not the only effect/affect the comedy produces, even though it is a significant ingredient of the emotional stance fostered by the genre. Eric Weitz, for instance, points both to a body of scholarship which presumes that the function of comedy is "to instruct" and to more recent arguments that call for exploring other facets of comedy, including its "spirited escape from harsher realities of corporeal existence" and the "psychic freedom with which it approaches the world" (9). Adoption comedy constellates and relies on these effects simultaneously as it tests the social consensus about kinship and reproduction. While plot conflicts may be resolved by affirming the social order that was disrupted yet survived, adoption comedy also indulges elements of what Andrew Horton describes as "pre-oedipal comedy"—a comedy where "wish fulfillment [and] dreams" escape the constraints of "parental or social hindrance" (10). These comedies end not in a "disavowal of any real disturbance" (King 8) but in a reality transformed by the social transgression. Social transformations are achieved through a "character's success" in fulfilling their "incredible fantasies" (Horton and Rapf 11), unlike in oedipal comedy (e.g., Shakespearean), which ends in "accommodation, compromise, social integration" (10) wherein the characters ultimately "must act like 'adults' to the degree of committing themselves to each other and thus to life within society" (11). In adoption comedies, secondary characters are often involved in pre-oedipal scenarios that are not neatly wrapped up in oedipal resolutions of the main plotline. Such incongruent elements are often perceived by the viewers and reviewers as unresolved storylines or superfluous characters since they cannot be fully assimilated in the normative narrative structure within the boundaries of a heterocoital plot. In other words, they are perceived as uncontainable narrative excess and their significance overlooked. Pre-oedipal storylines can be understood as serving to normalizing adoptive families by contrast (adoption is culturally queer but not *that* queer), and yet, such elements may also resist erasure as nonviable modes of being and may continue queering our thinking about kinship.

The Jerk is a film that can serve as a vivid example of comedy that results from "a sense of things being out of place, mixed up or not quite right," a departure from "'normal' routines of life of the social group in question" (King 5). In the film, Navin R. Johnson (Steve Martin) is a white adopted son of a Black sharecropper family in Mississippi. As an adoption story and a parody of rags-to-riches stories, *The Jerk* plays with stereotypes about race and class: Navin grows up poor, leaves home in search of fortune, strikes it big as an inventor, and then is destroyed by a lawsuit. The comedy in *The Jerk* is built around Navin's extreme naivete, which makes him socially awkward

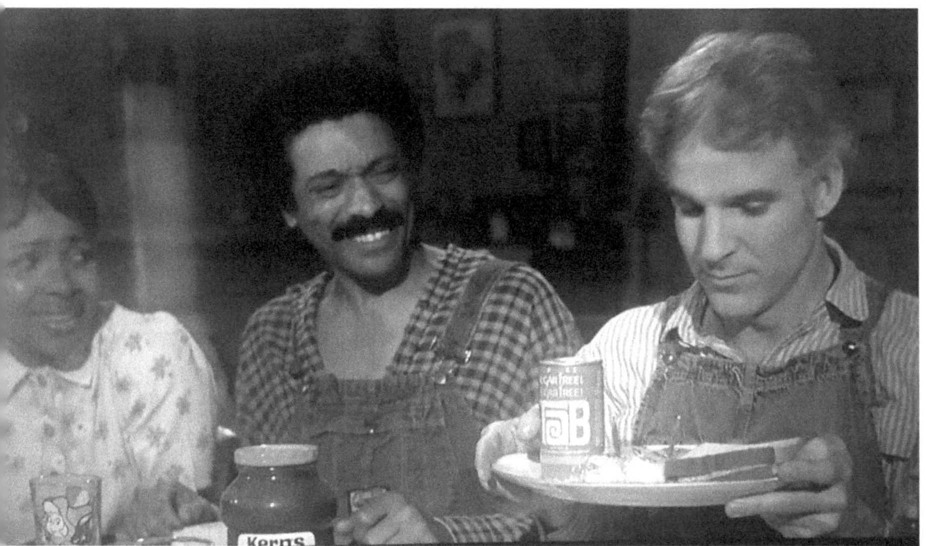

IGURE 3.1. Navin's birthday dinner in *The Jerk*. Universal Pictures, 1979.

and utterly clueless about the actual meaning of events in his life. The film opens up with homeless Navin talking to the camera-viewer about his story. He says, "It was never easy for me. I was born a poor Black child." His naivete is introduced at the beginning of the film as his total lack of awareness about being adopted, even though he is obviously white and the adoptive family attend to his difference by introducing elements of white culture into his life. For his birthday, his adoptive mother (Mabel King) makes a special treat, his "favorite meal"—tuna on white bread, a Tab, and Twinkies, while the whole family is eating collard greens (see figure 3.1). By showing Navin's preference for food culturally coded as "white" in the absence of his understanding that he is white, the film invokes the idea of race as difference at the genetic level. It is implied that he cannot fully belong with the Black family because he does not have the right nature to enjoy the adoptive family culture as his own. This idea is strengthened by Navin's lack of interest in the blues: the songs "depress" him, and when he tries to dance to the blues together with his family, his movements are awkward—he has no sense of the beat. His inability to participate in cultural practices coupled with his commitment to identifying as Black is construed as incongruent and comedic.

Knowledge of his adoption comes as a surprise to him. The withholding of adoption information from Navin and a lack of explanation of what is happening to him is yet another reversal of a recognizable cultural scenario done for a comedic effect. The lack of trust in the white family's ability to prepare a child to survive in racist society is transformed in the film into Navin's Black family not preparing him to use and enjoy his white privilege. His adoptive mother decides to tell him that he is adopted on his birthday, when Navin feels sad and overwhelmed during his birthday dinner. He rushes to his room and throws himself on the bed crying (the comedic effect is enhanced by his child-like behavior even though he looks like an adult man). His mother follows and asks, "Feeling different again, huh?" Navin answers, "It's like I don't fit in. Like I don't belong here." His mother explains that he is "old enough" to know that he is adopted and says they raised him "like you were one of us!" Navin is surprised, "You mean I'm gonna stay this color?" This exchange shows that he is not clueless about their difference, but he has no understanding of the ways culture connects genealogy to visual markers of race. Navin is waiting for nature to "catch up" and is clueless about the connection between heterocoital reproduction and biocultural traits that are used to establish one's belonging within a family and community. This naivete about reproduction is later underscored by his cluelessness about courtship rituals, sex, and what his "special purpose" (his penis) is for. He does not connect his race to his heterocoital origin and thus de-essentializes race by reversing the cultural understanding of it as grounded in "nature." He imagines it as a developmental trait acquired through nurture. By coupling the suggestion that Navin's whiteness is genetically coded with his expectation to eventually become Black, which denaturalizes race, *The Jerk* scrambles conventional ideas about reproduction and race and invites other ways of thinking about them.

As a solution to this situation, the plot follows a variation on the search and reunion scenario. Navin feels a connection to his "roots" when he hears an easy listening swing number played by a radio station in St. Louis. This music, culturally coded as white, speaks to him—he is dancing to its beat with abandon and is so excited by this sense of belonging that he wakes up the whole family to share his discovery. Soon after, he decides to leave home and travel to St. Louis to "be someone"—a typical aspiration of a young man, which, in this case, is inflected with an adoptee's need to reunite with his "nature." There is no biogenetic family to reunite with for Navin, though, and his origin search story is presented as a story of his attempt at a reunion with white privilege.

The adoptee's search for origins is thus presented as reestablishment of the naturalized connection between heterocoital origin and racialized class. But the film mocks this connection: having grown up "a poor Black child," Navin seems to have no idea of how to make use of his white privilege, which becomes another source of jokes in the film. When he is removed from his adoptive family, the world reads him as white, and much comedy is produced by his failure to perform entitled whiteness. He gladly works for meager pay at a gas station and is awed by the owner's offer to let him live in the broom closet, the entrance to which is through the restroom. In fact, he is excited even when he thinks his boss is suggesting he should live in the restroom itself. He speaks of his decoration plans for the place, using the vocabulary of upscale interior design—yet another joke underscoring the race-class incongruities he represents. Even after striking it rich, he struggles with communicating his status through his possessions. He buys expensive furnishings and a car that do not fit his modest-size suburban home. Only after he is reunited with the love of his life, Marie (Bernadette Peters), and they move to an over-the-top nouveau-riche mansion, his status as a rich white man is signaled, with her help, "adequately" and ridiculously. All the while, though, Navin identifies as Black. Before he leaves home, he earnestly takes the advice of his adoptive father (Richard Ward) not to "trust the whitey," even though he does not really know what that means and later does trust white people to help him, even as they take advantage of him. After he becomes rich, in a conversation about investment opportunities with some shady developers who share their plans to kick Black tenants out of their apartment complex, he yells at them, "*I*'m a n——!" and starts a fight. In the absence of genealogical connection to Blackness and given Navin's cultural behavior as white, his claim to Blackness seems to be grounded purely in his adoptive kinship. In other words, nature and culture are separated from kinship in Navin's thinking about his identity and place in the world.

Navin's success is presented simultaneously as earned by his ingenuity, accidental, and very likely assured by his white privilege. His idea of a modification to glasses is developed by Stan Fox (Bill Macy), a random customer he helps at the gas station, but his invention is not appropriated—an inversion of an exploited-minority-inventor story. He is found by Fox and given a hefty share of the profits. Navin does not have to work to maintain this wealth, but he is not in control of it. He receives the dividends from the venture, yet he is financially destroyed when the venture is mismanaged. His fortune is swiftly and accidentally taken away from him after a suit is filed by customers who have become cross-eyed due to using his invention. It may seem that this plot turn exploits the stereotype of a man who has grown up poor and cannot handle wealth responsibly, but it can also be read as mocking the randomness of his success, which is due to his assumed entitlement to white privilege. Another stereotype the film plays with is the "culture of poverty." It is subverted by showing Navin's adoptive family investing wisely the money he has been sending home. In this way, the family creates some wealth of their own, and after Navin loses everything, leaves Marie, and is homeless (for a day, even though he looks like he has been living in the streets for a while), his adoptive family comes to pick him up in a nice family car and wearing good clothes. They rescue him from the world where he tried to take his place as a white man and reunite him with his wife. When they all return to his adoptive home, the logic of class is subverted again. The family come back to a "bigger shack"; their house just grew in size, but it still looks the same. Even though they have money now, the family chooses to live the sharecroppers' culture, and the final scene of the film features the family on the porch of their shack, wearing old clothes, singing and dancing to the blues. By never connecting race and class definitively along the conventional cultural scripts for such correlations, the film uses adoption to comment on the arbitrariness of cultural markers of race and class, which ultimately puts in question the naturalized connection between them. *The Jerk* sets up play with cultural assumptions about race and class as biocultural categories by exploiting and simultaneously subverting race and class stereotypes.

The film does not completely abandon the heterocoital logic, though. The plot takes a turn and restores the heterocoital order by reconnecting Navin with his adoptive family through renaturing. In the final scene, Navin can dance to the beat, and he looks like he is enjoying the blues—a suggestion that his reunion with the adoptive family is marked by an emergence of a trait that was emphasized as genetically inaccessible to him earlier. The film suggests that Navin's newly found belonging with the adoptive family has been established because now his "nature" aligns with theirs enough to genuinely share cultural experiences with them. His growing up is marked by his growing into Blackness that he can now not only feel and claim as part of his identity but also perform more or less competently. Such renaturing simultaneously suggests the arbitrariness of assumptions about hereditary cultural transmission and reestablishes the importance of shared nature as a condition of belonging.

Adoptee renaturing as a way of belonging with the adoptive family becomes the basis of comedy in *Flirting with Disaster.* This film is a parody of the search and reunion narrative. Mel Coplin (Ben Stiller) is an adoptee whose story in the film begins with his inability to name his biological child unless he finds his birth parents. Unlike Navin, Mel sets out to reunite with actual people, not just the birth culture. He goes on a cross-country trip with his wife, Nancy (Patricia Arquette); his newborn son; and his adoption agent, Tina (Téa Leoni), who organizes and mishandles the reunion. The comedic effect is achieved by the reversal of the cultural expectation of "wholeness" and belonging that a reunion with the heterocoital origin can bring. The comedy of the film's middle is produced by misrecognitions—Mel reunites twice with people who are not his biological parents. In the process, he upends the lives of all the parents he attempts to reunite with, by endangering their possessions and exposing them to criminal liability. He troubles their kinship ties rather than enriching them, and even his reunion with the (finally) actual biological parents does not end with an instant connection and kinship tie reinstatement. His biological parents steal Mel's rental car and run for their lives without thinking about him after their drug running operation is accidentally exposed at the reunion dinner.

As adoption comedies often do, *Flirting* mocks the "ideology of resemblance" (Novy 77) that typically informs adoption reunions. The emotional peak of such narratives is typically the moment when biologically related children and parents meet for the first time and recognize each other through physical similarities (she has her grandmother's eyes!). Often, such ideology may present as genetic, traits that would typically be considered acquired through nurture. Like in the studies of twins separated at birth, who, after thirty years, find themselves both married to pilots, narratives of adoption reunions may produce heterocoital belonging through naturalization of sociocultural characteristics (he is a scientist, just like his biological father!). *Flirting* subverts such logic and shows Mel reinventing himself according to his assumed discovered heritage each time he meets a potential biological parent. The incongruity between his obvious physical and cultural difference from his prospective biological parents and his blind acceptance of them as such fuels the comedy. The first possible birth parent they meet is Valerie Swaney, a "Southern belle," a Reagan supporter, and a biological mother of tall blonde twin girls who look nothing like short, dark-haired Mel. He is "recognized" by them as possibly taking after their uncle to whom they refer as "a pervert." The physical difference between this genealogical line and Mel is obvious, but he is trying to fit in by showing acceptance of the culture, which is not his own: he, a liberal, expresses his approval of Reagan and accepts the idea of being a descendant of a Southern general (Nancy sings "Dixie" with Valerie). And yet, right after it seems that the family have bonded, to the degree that Valerie forgives Mel's accidental destruction of her glass figurine collection, Tina receives a call about a clerical mistake: Mel is not Valerie's son. The dissolution of belonging is immediate: the twins take back the T-shirt they gave Mel, and Valerie wants a compensation for her collection. This whiplash bonding and rejection puts in question the role of nature as an anchor for kinship ties. Even though the heterocoital status quo is restored with the discovery of Mel's heterocoital difference, the fact that his belonging was quickly forged with just a presumed heterocoital link suggests that "nature" does not have to be real to produce "real" kinship.

The film doubles down on this idea, and Mel's reunion with biological parents is delayed by one more false start. Mel's second attempt to establish heterocoital belonging is with Fritz Boudreau, a Michigan truck driver. By professing his lifelong wish to learn to drive a truck (which Nancy has never heard of), Mel is trying to be more like his father. The lesson ends with Mel backing the truck into a post office and an arrest of Fritz, who takes the blame. Before the accident, though, Fritz realizes that Mel might be a son of another man his mother met while she was his girlfriend. He figures it out by first noticing Mel's lack of resemblance to him and then by establishing a possibility of a genetic connection between Mel and Richard Schlichting because they are both scientists. The conflation of genetic and cultural transfer in this genealogical reasoning is yet another stab at the ideology of resemblance. The second unsuccessful attempt at a reunion builds up the viewers' expectations for Mel's "real" connection with the biological family, which, surely, should be different.

Indeed, during a reunion dinner with his biological parents, Mel finds out that he and Richard are both scientists. Richard says, "The genetic connection, right?" (105). Mary, the biological mother, shares that Lonnie, their younger son and Mel's biological brother, "never had interest in science," which provokes Lonnie's "What is this supposed to mean?" (105). What it means is that heterocoital logic can be deployed strategically and post-factum to legitimize or question a kinship tie. Mel and Lonnie's relationship questions the assumed link between genetic connection and familial feeling as well. The original film script states that the only visible genetic resemblance between family members is between Mel and Lonnie: they are "stunned at the resemblance" when they first see each other (102). Yet, the resemblance results in sibling rivalry at best. Mel finds Lonnie creepy, and Lonnie feels defensive since his parents like Mel "better because he's more like [them]" (111). In fact, Lonnie, who participates in the family's drug-dealing, seems to "take after" his parents more convincingly than Mel. He refuses to engage with Mel and tries to poison him with LSD. Mel feels ambivalent about his biological parents and balks at the information about their parental neglect and their lack of remorse about it: Mary reveals that she was taking LSD when pregnant with him and jokes that they were relieved when he came out with just one head. In the end, Mel feels a stronger sense of belonging with his neurotic, law-abiding adoptive parents. The film, which disrupts the idea of biocultural reproduction through Mel's misrecognitions, disrupts it again by renaturing Mel into the neuroticism of his adoptive family. Culture is thus imagined as both heterocoitally transmitted and not, and the film plays with the conflation of genetic and cultural transfer just enough to blur the line between nature and culture and to naturalize cultural categories. In this way, *Flirting*, like *The Jerk*, extends the assumption of naturalized transfer of culture into cultural transfer of nature and shows that heterocoital kinship ideas continue to inform belonging even in the absence of heterocoital link.

The framing of the film reflects this reinstatement of the role of heterocoital reproduction in imagining family. The importance of the heterocoital nature-culture link is established from the start, as Mel connects his own heterosexual and heterocoital futurity to being raised by biological parents or at least to knowing who they are. He needs to know his origin in order to understand himself and be able to produce his futurity: specifically, to name his own child. His inability to name his son unless he reconnects with the birth parents signals his belief that he is a link in a genealogical chain. He thinks it is his responsibility to reproduce his biological line of descent through a cultural gesture of giving his child a name used in the family. Without his origin knowledge, he is "distracted," "a little unsteady," and "preoccupied." Yet, Mel's reflection on his lack of knowledge about his biological parents undermines the heterocoital logic. He is trying to imagine what his birth parents might be, and his voice-over reflection is followed by jump cuts between images of "prospective" (6) parents: a "smart" rich woman, or a "stupid" rich woman, or a poor woman with a heart of gold, or an angry poor woman; then we see images of possible fathers of all sorts, including an itinerant person rooting through trash. Mel is trying to imagine his parents as couples—"They had to hook up in order to have me, right?" (6). One of these couplings includes two women, which opens up kinship possibilities beyond the normative heterocoital family. "Anything is possible," he says (6). He imagines that if he were raised by "at least one of [his] real parents" (6), he could have a totally different life (we get images of his potential heterosexual couplings). The peculiar conclusion that "anything is possible" ignores the possibility that some details about his heterocoital origin could be at least partially divined from the way he is now. He assumes that by knowing his biological parents he will know himself, but there is no assumption that by knowing himself he could predict what his biological parents were like. He seems to believe that the adoptive family's nurture and culture have "substituted" nature to the point that it needs to be "relearned" through a reunion with the biological line of descent. In Mel's mind, while nature is an elemental "ingredient" of who one really is and a guarantor of futurity, it is simultaneously presented as easily erasable, a complete unknown in the absence of knowledge about one's heterocoital genitors. Through showing Mel fixated on biological parents as determinant of his futurity, the film stresses the importance of heterocoital origin to one's identity. Yet, at the same time, by presenting Mel as easily adapting to any possibility of heterocoital origin and unable to divine it based on his own identity, *Flirting* introduces the idea that futurity is pliable and a child could be a conduit of any culture.

The film challenges heterocoital logic also through secondary plotlines that involve queer characters. In addition to Mel's imagining a possibility of being raised by two women, the middle of *Flirting* brings up other forms of queer kinship and reproduction. On their last leg of the reunion trip to New Mexico to meet the Schlichtings, Mel, Nancy, and Tina are accompanied by the FBI agents who handled Mel's destruction of the post office—a same-sex couple. One of them, Tony (Josh Brolin), is bisexual and an old flame of Nancy's. At a catch-up dinner, she invites him and his boyfriend along on a whim, triggered by Mel's suspected interest in Tina. She doesn't expect them to take the invitation seriously, but Tony and Richard (Paul Harmon) show up at the airport. Tony has an obvious interest in Nancy's baby—he has been trying to convince Richard to adopt and is hoping that being around the baby and Tina, an adoption agency worker, may help. At the end of the film, after the Schlichtings run away and Mel rescues his adoptive parents from jail with the help of Tony and Richard, the whole group has their picture taken on the steps of the police station. While setting up for the photo, Tony and Richard discuss adoption possibilities with Tina, who suggests an alternative option: asking a lesbian couple to participate in heterocoital reproduction and then "share" the child (138). The context in which the photo is taken thus focuses the viewers' attention on the adoptive family reunion against the background of nontraditional kinship, especially given the absence of Mel's biological family in it. Mel's adoption story follows a familiar cultural script for the adoptive family as an imitation of the biological, nuclear one. Ultimately, Mel recognizes his adoptive parents as his "real" parents, while the birth family who have made their appearance to make his heterocoital futurity possible (he can name his child now) flee across the border not to bother anyone again.

But the family photo scene is not the film's ending, even though it looks like one (reunion documentaries often close with a family photo that reflects the family configuration in which the adoptee places themselves as the outcome of the search). While the opening sequence of the film destabilizes the heterocoital link between nature and culture even as it establishes Mel's need to find his biological parents, and the middle challenges cultural scripts of reprosexuality, the "happy ending" doubles down on reconfirming heterocoital ideology. The very final sequence of the film features a series of scenes in which couples are in bed, having or trying to have sex. In all these instances, sex is interrupted by children: the Coplins have to babysit for Nancy and Mel, and their sex is interrupted by the baby crying; the Schlichtings are interrupted by their son Lonnie rummaging through the drawers in their bedroom looking for weed; Paul and Tony are trying to have sex next to a bassinette with a (somehow procured) baby inside but cannot move past negotiating where to put the baby and Richard's gun. The scene featuring a very pregnant Tina leaving her apartment to meet her blind date after she puts out a cigarette also suggests that her baby might be in the way of her plans. These scenes of nonreproductive senior sex, gay sex, and a single unwed smoking mother dating while pregnant are framed by shots of Nancy and Mel in bed—the normalized heterosexual reproductive couple. Their heterosexual desire is allowed to unfold to its heterocoital conclusion (nothing distracts them), suggesting the possibility of another round of reproduction. While nonnormative sex and reproduction are happening around Mel and Nancy, their story of a heterosexual married couple who have reproduced and may continue to reproduce heterocoitally becomes the frame and focus of the film.

The Jerk and *Flirting with Disaster* are comedies that end with wish-fulfillment of the adoptive family and the adoptee aligned: the adoptive family is reunited, and the adoptee has explored their birth culture or met with their birth family but has not felt their pull enough to separate from the adoptive family. In both films, the adoptee's belonging with the adoptive family and culture is imagined as renaturing of the adoptee, who is reincorporated into the adoptive family through reinventing cultural belonging as a genetic connection. In this way, both adoptive and heterocoital family are positioned as acceptable forms of kinship as long as they do not visibly clash with heterocoital cultural scripts. And, ultimately, Mel's own heterocoital reproduction assures normative futurity and makes his adoption an exception in his genealogical line.

Fakin' da Funk and *Catfish in Black Bean Sauce* negotiate adoption in similar ways, but they portray transracial adoption that excludes white family members and white communities. By bracketing out whiteness and decentering the idea that transnational and transracial adoption is predominantly the domain of white parents, these films explore the flow of power through kinship formations in the context of relationships between minority cultures. Even though whiteness may remain an implicit point of reference in the cultural power hierarchy (e.g., the discourses by which minority culture defends itself from appropriation are informed by responses to the dominant culture), *Fakin'* and *Catfish* specifically show how minority cultures may negotiate nonheterocoital belonging and kinship through cultural appropriation and assimilation discourses. *Fakin'* features a Chinese adoptee[2] raised by a Black family, and *Catfish* is a story of two Vietnamese children adopted by the family of a

2. It is not clear if Julian is a domestic or transnational adoptee, since the film never gives us his pre-adoption story.

Black US military officer. In both films, the humor is based on the disruption of the assumed nature-culture transfer: an Asian body is reproducing Black culture, and an Asian adoptee ignores, misrecognizes, or, in the eyes of their community, fails to "naturally" connect to biological parents, same-race people, or culture. Like the comedies discussed at the beginning of this chapter, *Fakin'* and *Catfish* imagine renaturing through cultural assimilation as a condition of belonging in adoption. Yet they also reveal that the key to such renaturing is not only an expert performance of the "right" culture by the adoptee, but the family's and the larger community's acceptance of this performance as sanctioned and genuine.

Even though heterocoital, nuclear, middle-class family ideology may still be operative as the norm, the absence of visible whiteness in these transracial adoption narratives complicates both the assumption that children of color are better off if adopted by same-race or white parents and the idea that transracial adoption is a form of colonization. Transracial and transnational adoption by white parents is sometimes understood through a postcolonial framework as the child's assimilation into an "ours but not quite" position of the colonized that entails a loss of a genuine connection to birth culture and to "who they are." This framework demands that the adoptee's connection to the origin culture be restored so they could resist this form of oppression.[3] Some accounts understand minority transracial adoptive kinship in relation to kinship and adoption norms grounded in the cultural practices of the dominant white middle-class culture that defines kinship norms. In the case of the US, for instance, Rachel Rains Winslow and Kori Graves have shown that the logic of placements in postwar transnational adoptions was defined by domestic racial hierarchies of the time.[4] Such frameworks may be helpful to understanding some specifics of adoption negotiations in *Fakin'* and *Catfish.* For example, transnational adoption by an African American family may be

3. This approach is critiqued by John McLeod. See McLeod (2018) for an account of postcolonial studies' engagement with the subject of adoption, including his discussion and critique of Pal Ahluwalia's "Negotiating Identity: Postcolonial Ethics and Transnational Adoption."

4. Winslow's analysis of claims to Black, Asian, and especially multi-race adoptees by prospective adoptive parents and communities in the US reveals a belief that race and "culture" of a child should match. More interestingly, her analysis of postwar transnational adoptions reveals simultaneous colorblindness and insistence on the Black-white distinction characteristic of the US society at work in discussions of which children belong where and with what kinds of families. In particular, the instance of whitewashing of Korean adoptees by the Holts, who "identified their adopted children as Americans" (88), that is, denied them any involvement with Korean culture, with the simultaneous insistence on placing Black Korean children with Black families reveals the peculiarities of the American racial hierarchies and points to the body of an Asian adoptee as a site of struggle over cultural reproduction. *Fakin'* may lend itself to a reading that would see the Asian adoptee as "blackwashed," which establishes African American culture as dominant and worth assimilating to.

understood as part of the civil rights "struggle to obtain equality" by claiming the power "to interven[e] in complicated domestic and foreign affairs" (Graves 16, 5). And the Asian adoptee's negotiations of belonging could be seen as negotiations with a culture that had a long tradition of imagining Asian immigrants as not able or willing to "assimilate into American culture or society" (Graves 15). *Fakin'* and *Catfish,* however, subvert the logic of the power structure in which "international adoption [is] the unequivocal domain of white parents" and "assimilability into whiteness [is] the standard by which multiracial children [are] measured" (Winslow 178, 158) by presenting a transracial and transnational adoption scenarios in which an Asian adoptee becomes a site of a somewhat different cultural negotiation because whiteness is bracketed out.[5] Such inversion puts focus on the relationship between African American and Asian communities and kin. In this case, understanding the use of culture in negotiations of transracial belonging may not follow the logic of colonizer-colonized or white-Black power structures, as we are looking at the relationships between two cultures that would be considered "oppressed" in relation to the dominant one. In this case, the concept of cultural appropriation as well as Thi Nguyen and Strohl's account of intimacy and cultural belonging may help us better understand Asian adoptees' negotiation of belonging in Black families and communities as they are represented in *Fakin'* and *Catfish.*

As other adoption narratives, these films show how an assumed link between reproduction and culture transfer makes adoption a situation of a cultural encounter and struggle and the adoptee a contested site of cultural reproduction. Inclusion of an Asian adoptee in a Black community and family raises the question of what culture the Asian body will reproduce in this context. Storylines that decenter white culture and feature Black adoptive parents place Black culture in the position of power, and the Asian adoptee needs to define their stance in relation to Blackness. This situation makes the biocultural clash caused by adoption more apparent, since a minority target culture that is both culturally distinct and less socially privileged displaces a default norm for assimilation, which is to say, whiteness that is perceived as culturally neutral, normative, and racially unmarked. In addition to assimilation and origin recovery that are typically negotiated in adoption narratives, in this case the adoptee has to also navigate accusations of cultural appropriation, "a complementary opposite" to assimilation as a mode of cultural transmission

5. It is possible to say that it remains present in the assumption of the nuclear family's primacy. In *Fakin',* the family of the adoptee becomes single-mother, but by widowhood, and it is a nuclear family at the time of adoption. Other forms of family, e.g., the extended multigenerational family, are not front and center.

(Ziff and Rao 5). Ziff and Rao suggest that "differential access to power" (5) determines how we view instances of culture transfer, and "depending on whether the subjectivity of the receiver of culture is identified as being from a dominant or a subordinate group" (5), cultural transmission can be "read as appropriation or assimilation" (6). The adoptee's negotiation of belonging as power negotiation between two minority cultures is especially noticeable in *Fakin'* since the Asian adoptee's attempts to establish his belonging in Los Angeles's South Central are happening against the implied backdrop of postriot tensions between Asian and Black communities. His expert and genuine cultural performance of Black masculinity is initially perceived by the community of South Central as cultural appropriation, the kind that Nguyen and Strohl would consider a threat to "group intimacy" rather than a breach of "property rights" or "harm" (981). Their account of intimacy explains belonging in a minority group as a result of daily cultural practices that "generate relations of group intimacy, which can ground certain prerogatives in much the same way that interpersonal intimacy can" (981). The established boundaries depend on "what the group decides together" rather than prior precedents and legal discourses (981). Within such an account, "oppression" of a minority culture is a condition "that gives the prerogatives of intimacy heightened normative importance" (990). Therefore, the adoptee in *Fakin'* is challenged to convince the Black community that his performance of Black culture is not a cultural appropriation, as he earns the right to participate in communal intimacy.

In *Fakin'*, the adoptee's belonging in a Black family and larger community is negotiated twice: first, at the time of his adoption as a baby in Atlanta, and then, after his relocation from Atlanta, where he first grows up, to LA's South Central. The film opens with a scene at a Black church. The camera follows people who are entering the church and then zooms in on the choir. We see Julian Lee (Dante Basco) singing with abandon next to two young boys, who are Black. After the hymn is done, the minister delivers a sermon as a send-off to the Lee family—Julian; his mother, Annabelle (Pam Greer); and his younger brother, the Lees' biological son, Perry (Rashaan Nall). They are moving from Atlanta to LA following the death of the father, the former minister of the church. The incongruity of Julian's placement within a Black community is further explained through voice-over. Julian tells the story of his adoption, intercut with scenes that show the moments of adoption and his childhood. Julian directly addresses the audience and acknowledges that the viewers may be wondering how he ended up in this context. He says that it was a "mistake," but not a "love child or something"—"this mistake was a whole lot different." In fact, the mistake was due to the racially ambiguous last name of Annabelle and Joe—Lee, which can belong to racially diverse ethnicities. When a nurse comes out and asks who Annabelle Lee is (leave it to Poe to evoke the possible "whiteness" of the name), he is surprised to see a Black couple. The nurse says, "But you are Black!" to which Annabelle, angered and confused by his statement, replies, "And you are white!" The nurse snorts as he hands the baby over, and the Lees understand the reason for his remark as they pull the blanket off the baby's face. An Asian baby is looking back at them. This mistaken identity scenario is echoed in the secondary storyline of the Chinese exchange student May-Lee (Margaret Cho), who is placed with a South Central Black family, instead of a Canadian exchange student, Marilyn Lee. The confusions based on a family name that exists in different cultures, even though its origins are situated in specific ethnic contexts, destabilize the last name as a cultural marker of racially homogenous heterocoital reproduction and turn it into a loaded metaphor for non-heterocoital kinship.

Julian's introduction to the Lees begins with a conflict between his adoptive parents about his belonging in a Black family. When they see Julian for the first time, Joe (Ernie Hudson) says, "This is not the baby we ordered" and insists they cannot keep the baby because he belongs with "folks of his own kind." Annabelle, on the other hand, says that all the child needs is a loving home. The terms of cultural negotiation are introduced when Joe connects biological origin to culture while Annabelle's understanding of kinship denaturalizes it. Joe is wondering if Annabelle can make Chinese food to feed the child, to which Annabelle responds, "who says he has to eat Chinese food?" "What about chopsticks?" "We don't have any." "Well, that's my point!" Joe connects cultural differences to belonging in larger communities as he wonders, "Think about what folks are gonna say later on in life: a Chinese kid growing up in the hood?" His concern is echoed by Julian, who is wondering in the voice-over about the reaction of the Chinese family that received a Black baby—"Can you imagine!?" The blunt, insensitive discussion of adoption issues (commercialization, adoption agencies' errors, racial matching) that are typically silenced or hedged is a hallmark of the comedy genre, which modulates the impact of bluntness on the viewer through comedic performances. The uncertainty about Julian's belonging is processed through humor that nevertheless invites to engage with serious matters.

Julian's own negotiation of belonging begins with a childish, overstated performance of Blackness. A cut between two scenes with Julian at elementary-school age contrasts the ways Joe and Julian deal with his racial difference. One of the scenes shows Joe practicing his sermon in front of the bathroom mirror as he shaves. He says, "It matters not the color of the skin," when little Julian peeks in. Joe asks if his son wants to know what this sermon is about, but Julian rolls his eyes and leaves. Joe sighs, "I guess, you are not going to be following in my footsteps." He expresses disillusionment in his adopted son's potential to contribute to father-son intimacy by continuing the professional and genealogical line. In this way, he connects belonging and intimacy to heterocoital genealogy: the color of the skin may not matter, but biogenetic connection does. This scene is cut to a classroom, where Julian, pacing in front of the blackboard, preaches racial harmony. He *is* following in Joe's footsteps by taking interest in preaching. Mimicking his father's speech cadences, he says, "I pray for the day when you love me as much as I love you all." A white girl responds, "I love you," which Julian answers with a long tirade about his rejection of Black and white interracial intimacy: "I don't like cream in my coffee"; "This ain't jungle fever, baby." The comedic effect is achieved by the discrepancy between the mixed meanings of the word "love" as well as between Julian's beliefs, the way he looks, and the family he belongs with. It seems he does not understand the way he may be seen by his community and larger racial structure. He refuses to see the color of his skin, while underscoring the girl's, and draws on Black-versus-white cultural scripts of racial separation in intimate relationships in order to assert his Black identity. With an emphatic expression of cultural values common in his community, Julian aims to overcome the biogenetic difference signaled by his body. He does not remain stuck in non-awareness like Navin in *The Jerk*, though. His deliberate choice to be or stay Black as he is growing up is revealed when he is displaced from the community that recognizes his belonging.

While Julian is accepted in Atlanta as a known member of a Black family, when they have to move to South Central LA, he clashes with the community there. The mismatch between his body and the culture it performs is jarring to those unfamiliar with his life story, and he is seen as a poser and a cultural appropriator. In LA, he is expected to be "authentically" Asian, and his expert performance of Black culture baffles and angers. The narrative situates his negotiation of belonging in South Central on the basketball court and within his relationship with a young woman he wants to date. The scene of his introduction to the new community shows that he is perceived as an identity threat by the young Black men he engages with on the court. They approach Julian and his brother, Perry, hoping that Perry can play. They speak to Julian in broken English, taking him to be an Asian immigrant, and are surprised when he responds in fluent Black English. While they are impressed at first and show respect for the "little flavor" he has, they get defensive when he turns out to be really good at basketball. They have an argument over a pass, and one of the young men, Brandon (Duane Martin), gets into an altercation with Julian during which he calls Julian both a "Chinaman" and the n-word. The exchange quickly becomes comical because they can no longer track who called whom what, and at some point, Brandon complains that Julian called him a "Chinaman." This confusion, although presented as funny, signals a potential threat of cultural appropriation represented by the incongruity of Julian's expert performance of Black culture that could be recognized as authentic but for his embodiment. His hybridity compromises the identity boundary that has been set through cultural practices as a matter of claiming cultural power by restricting participation of outsiders in such practices. The way Julian *is* challenges the community to decide whether he can be allowed to engage in its cultural practices or whether what he is doing is cultural appropriation against which the community must defend itself.[6] Further development of the scene connects the threat of cultural appropriation to a reproductive script. The argument between young men is interrupted by the arrival of girls, and Julian is immediately attracted to one of them, Karyn (Tatyana Ali). He is called out on his attempts to smooth-talk her by other young men, who use his racial difference to signal who is "allowed" to date Black girls. By shouting, "What are you looking at? She ain't your type," and suggesting he should keep "breaded shrimp in [his] pants," they assert their identity and draw reproductive boundaries against racial outsiders—the way Julian did in his elementary school classroom when he was responding to the white girl's "I love you." At the same time, they are mocking his hybridity ("What's next? Dude's gonna star in Alex Haley's new movie, *Ginseng Roots*") by casting it as freakish ("Why are you here?"; "I live here. I belong here"; "No you belong in Rikki Lake").

Acceptance eventually comes to Julian both on the basketball court and in his relationship with Karyn. The community's perception of his performances of Black culture changes from seeing them as cultural appropriation to their acceptance of them as evidence of his assimilation. Such reframing redefines "power relationships" implied in culture transfer processes (Ziff and Rao 5) and makes it possible for the community to extend group intimacy to Julian when it becomes known that he is adopted by a Black family and that he has experienced life the way a Black person might. When Brandon and Karyn learn about Julian's adoptive family, they accept Julian as a friend and a boyfriend. Brandon witnesses Julian's decision to risk his own future in order to

6. Transracial adoptions, both domestic and transnational, often disrupt established cultural ideas and scripts that maintain racial, ethnic, and national boundaries. The disruptions reveal the purposes of such ideas and scripts, as well as the purposes of adoption and other forms of kinship, in drawing such boundaries. For discussions of this subject in CAS, see the work of Eleana Kim, Kim Park Nelson, Kim McKee, Sara Dorow, Dorothy Roberts, Kori Graves, Margaret Jacobs, Karen Balcom, and others.

save his adoptive brother, Perry, from the influence of the local "community organizer" and drug lord, Frog. Even though Julian's racial difference and its rejection by the community make Perry distance himself from his adoptive brother, Julian agrees to do a drug run for Frog in order to sever Perry's connection with Frog's circle. Beyond just the fact of his kinship with the adoptive Black family, Julian acts as a "real" brother to Perry by putting himself in danger to protect Perry from the drug dealer. In the eyes of Brandon, this behavior "proves" Julian's kinship with a Black brother and makes him a genuine culture performer rather than a poser. Brandon admits that he had been thinking of Julian as a Michael-Jordan-obsessing cultural appropriator until he found out about what Julian had done for his family. Julian's belonging is also confirmed by Perry, who says in response to Brandon's question of whether Julian is his adopted brother, "No, man. He is my brother." As an intimacy-establishing gesture, Brandon shares with Julian the story of his own brother's shooting and says, "You and me, we are alike." They bond over loving brothers who lived through archetypal community experiences. Adoption is erased in this act of bonding, and same-race belonging is suggested through an assertion of biogenetic relatedness.

Brandon's personal acceptance of Julian extends to communal intimacy, which is publicly confirmed on basketball court. To help Julian, Brandon challenges Frog's entourage to a game of hoops: if Julian's team wins, he and his brother do not owe Frog anything. Brandon's offer shows his confidence in Julian's skills and intimate knowledge about Julian's basketball competence, which may not be known to the outsiders. Brandon shows up to make his offer when Frog is styling Julian to look like a Japanese tourist in order to avoid suspicion during his drug run. Frog is putting glasses, a baseball hat, a messenger bag, and a camera on frustrated Julian. After Brandon's suggestion is accepted, Julian tears off his "costume," throws it to the ground, and says, "Let's do this!" He is rejecting the vision of himself as a foreigner or outsider and claims his belonging to Black culture by asserting cultural competence that Frog's entourage would not expect from an Asian young man. The game follows the typical underdog scenario: Julian's team loses at first and he gets injured, but at the last moment, after Perry shows up, Julian shoots a three-pointer, wins the game, and Frog's team retreats in defeat. Karyn and Annabelle are also in the audience, witnessing Julian's victory with other people from the community. Thus, in front of everyone, Julian's belonging and the permission to reproduce Black culture are confirmed. Allegorically, the game also decides which Black culture and kinship Julian and his brother are going to reproduce: the ersatz "family" of the drug gang or his *real* adoptive family and the good people of his community.

The permission to reproduce culture is supported by the permission to engage in a heterosexual, potentially reproductive romantic relationship with a Black girl. Julian's acceptance as part of the community also leads to his acceptance for "who he is" by Karyn. While initially Karyn sees Julian as exotic, in the end, she accepts him as authentically (culturally) Black. Karyn is interested in Japanese culture, and she initially misreads Julian as an expert on any Asian culture. It becomes clear, however, when they go out to a Japanese restaurant, that he has no knowledge of Japanese or Chinese languages or cultures. Karyn is wearing a cheongsam-like dress and is on friendly terms with the chef, who graciously treats her pan-Asian cultural confusion and possible appropriation as a "beneficial cultural exchange" (Nguyen and Strohl, 986). The irony of multiple "confusions" about cultural boundaries is underscored when Karyn says she wants to go to Japan and Julian says he wants to go to Africa to find out about his roots. Karyn's stance toward "foreign" cultures defines the way she sees Julian as trying to be who he is not. While Karyn tells him that she accepts him for who he is, she actually fails to see his biocultural hybridity and breaks up with him because "if [he is] not going to be real with [her], then [she doesn't] think [they] should be seeing each other." Julian responds by asserting his Blackness, "I'm Black. I'm proud of being Black, and I'm more Black than you'll ever be." While Karyn's reaction is informed by biocultural consistency bias, Julian points to class-specific cultural practices as racial markers as he delivers an implicit critique of Karyn's class status. This critique also shows Julian's understanding of himself as a member of a community that negotiates belonging of its members based on group intimacy. He aims to carry out such a negotiation with Karyn by doubting whether her experiences are shared by the group to which she denies him acceptance. Karyn, whose appearance and heterocoital origin make her secure in her racial identity, is surprised by what she takes to be an accusation of being disloyal to Black culture. Her response implies that heterocoital origin is her guarantee of acceptance: "I don't need to live in the hood to be Black." Her lack of knowledge about his adoption leads them to an impasse and prevents her from seeing his "authentic" self because she cannot yet see a reason to revise the assumption of biocultural belonging.

Julian's eventual acceptance by Karyn is simultaneously a legitimization of Julian's reproductive future as a conduit of Black culture. In the making-up scene, Karyn says, "It's what on the inside that counts" and suggests they go out for some soul food instead of Chinese or Japanese. Their getting back together ends with a tumble from the couch onto the floor—a suggestion of sex which confirms that Karyn finally accepts Julian as a romantic and potentially reproductive partner who identifies as Black. But is he accepted as "who he is," a biocultural hybrid? Karyn finds out that Julian has not told her he was adopted because of a painful past experience. Annabelle tells her that Julian's ex-girlfriend's parents broke them up after they found out his family was Black. Annabelle explains, "That's when he made the vow that people are going to accept him for who he is." Julian seems to assert the complexity of his biocultural makeup, but the film shows that such hybridity may not guarantee belonging with the group in which he seeks acceptance. His belonging in South Central is acknowledged when he is seen as "engaging in intimate acts" within a kinship structure that is embedded in the Black community (Nguyen and Strohl 991). Shared community intimacy becomes possible not only through his actions or archetypal group experiences but also because Julian is a son and a brother of a Black family. Once this becomes known, his cultural Blackness becomes acceptable and the difference of his embodiment is minimized. But when he is seen as equal to a biological family member, his adoptee status is minimized, and his hybridity is obscured. Such necessarily reductive logic of belonging is also present in the story involving his ex-girlfriend. The rejection of Julian as a potential boyfriend of a presumably Asian or white young woman happens when it becomes known that his family is Black. Culture alone seems to be insufficient for rejection, but once Julian's adoptive family identity is revealed, his embodiment does not seem to be enough. He becomes unacceptable to the ex-girlfriend's family when they learn that he is tied to a Black family by kinship. In these negotiations, culture and nature seem to take a back seat to known kinship ties which have the power to redefine how someone's embodiment and cultural identification are read.

Unlike many adoption narratives, *Fakin'* does not raise the issue of Julian's lack of connection to Chinese culture as an injustice. He is not interested in the pursuit of origin knowledge and expresses no need to "reconnect" with his birth culture beyond borrowing a Chinese phrase book from May-Lee, the Chinese exchange student, in order to impress Karyn. Julian's divestment from his originary culture means that the adoptive Black culture is not hybridized by his presence. The threat of community hybridization he presents is externalized and displaced onto May-Lee's storyline, which shows her engaged in a "mutually beneficial cultural exchange" with the Black community (Nguyen and Strohl 986). The narrative solves the double bind adoptees find themselves in ("adoptee, know thy origin" vs. "be like us to be our own") by having each of these two cultural demands fulfilled by a different character. Julian's perceived foreignness is set off against May-Lee's literal one in order to create a gradation of belonging and portray him as "one of our own" compared to the "honorary stranger" membership of May-Lee. The film imagines their relationship with the Black culture as assimilation of Julian and cultural exchange with May-Lee. While she starts out as a clueless foreigner, eventually she is symbolically adopted by her host family and romantically involved with Brandon. After some time, her fear of living "in the hood" is gone to the extent that she refuses to either live with a Chinese American family or go back home as her parents want. She acquires some Black culture knowledge, but she is also told, "you do not have to act Black." This statement is a recognition and acceptance of what she is—Chinese—but also a setting of a boundary that limits the terms of her belonging to being an honorary stranger who will eventually leave. Over the course of May-Lee's stay in South Central, we can see her improve her dancing skills, learn to drive Brandon's lowrider, and give directions like a local to an Asian man who seems to have just arrived. In turn, she has some impact on the local community. She helps Brandon become more open, and one day she leads a crowd of neighbors in a session of tai chi.

The community seems culturally influenced by May-Lee's symbolic adoption more than by Julian's literal one. This exchange is possible due to her imprecise cultural performances, her foreign citizenship and kinship, as well as her accent, which mark as safe her limited expertise on Black culture. The Black community's participation in Chinese culture together with May-Lee is not perceived as a threat of cultural erosion in the way Julian's seamless assimilation and refusal to accept that he is Asian is. His visible hybridity has to be handled through a belonging narrative that minimizes his attachment to the Chinese culture and portrays him as fully assimilated into Black culture. Ultimately, both Julian's and May-Lee's storylines portray Black culture as not only socially powerful as a result of its resistance to appropriation claims and drawing boundaries against strangers but also as one worth assimilating into and worthy of cultural exchange with. Julian's literal and May-Lee's symbolic adoptions suggest that nontraditional kinship provides a way for a minority culture to claim power by opening its boundaries and allowing strangers to participate in the culture on its own terms. At the same time, *Fakin'* suggests that to address the threat of cultural identity erosion (a common concern for nondominant cultures), the logic of such empowerment demands of someone who wants to belong either a full assimilation and participation in drawing boundaries against strangers or staying at a respectful distance of cultural exchange.

Catfish in Black Bean Sauce, another film featuring Asian adoptees and African American adoptive parents, introduces the adoptee's birth culture into the narrative in a more visible way and explores possibilities for cultural acceptance of the adoptee's biocultural complexity further. *Catfish,* similar to

Fakin', uses the bifurcation of storylines as a narrative mechanism to separate cultures in relation to which adoptees have to situate themselves. In this case, splitting the adoptee's double bind between two sibling adoptees makes it possible to show variations on adoptees' positionality in relation to their birth culture. We see siblings Mai (Lauren Tom) and Dwayne (Chi Muoi Lo) engage with their adoption history in different ways. While Mai is married to a Vietnamese American and is searching for her biological parents, Dwayne is more concerned about fitting into his adoptive Black culture than reconnecting with his Vietnamese origin. Dwayne identifies as Black and is confident in his culture performance yet struggling with insecurities grounded in racialized stereotypes about his embodiment. This struggle affects his romance with Nina (Sanaa Lathan), a young Black woman. His doubts about belonging in the Black community are explored mostly through this relationship. The primary storyline of the film is Dwayne's, and, ultimately, he finds his identity as culturally Black with enough knowledge of and openness to his birth culture to satisfy the common cultural script of the adoptee's belonging. Mai's is a foil to Dwayne's storyline. Her husband is her racial match, and she is focused on creating a visibly continuous genealogical line by bringing her birth mother to live with them. She initiates the film's conflict by finding the birth mother and bringing Thanh (Kieu Chinh) over to the US, which causes a rift between her and Dolores (Mary Alice), the adoptive mother. At the end of the film, she is reconciled with both mothers, but the shape of her household obscures her biocultural complexity, while Dwayne, who chooses a Black woman as his partner, seems oriented toward reproducing his. Following the logics of their respective belonging processes, the comedic elements associated with Mai's story focus on disrupting and inverting typical narratives of genetic certainty (she fails to recognize her birth mother at the airport, twice), while Dwayne's storyline builds comedy around uncertainties caused by clashes between his cultural expression and embodiment.

In contrast to Julian, Dwayne is portrayed as not-so-seamlessly integrated into Black culture. Dwayne's performance of Blackness is anchored in his speech, and he is presented as simultaneously unaware of how his cultural expression is read by others outside of his family circle and acutely aware of his potential inadequacies encoded in racialized stereotypes of masculinity. The opening scene of the film shows Dwayne playing cards with his adoptive parents and discussing the cat that Henry (Paul Winfield), his adoptive father, volunteered to take in at their pastor's request. Dolores wants to find a home for this cat, but Dwayne is adamant about not wanting it. He says, "Don't even try it," and this is the first time we hear him speaking in an accent intended to sound "Black." The family are talking about why they can't keep the cat and who else might take it,[7] and Dwayne points out that "something ain't right about that cat." Dolores explains that the cat is blind, but to Dwayne the cat's oddity is her misidentification with what she is not. He says, "I mean, look at her—she thinks she is human," pointing at the cat, who is sleeping on her back. The opening credits roll over the cat exploring the backyard, but it looks like she is not blind and knows what she is doing.

The cat who acts like a human and seems to be blind is introduced as a metaphor for the biocultural complexity of Dwayne, who can be read by people outside of his family as acting strange when he is performing Black speech and as lacking awareness about the perceived clash between his embodiment and his cultural performance. At the same time, the sequence of scenes that follows the opening shows Dwayne acutely aware of his potential inadequacies when he compares himself to a Black man. In the scene that follows the cat discussion, Dwayne is shown planning to propose to Nina, but his attempt is thwarted by his roommate Michael's arrival. Michael introduces his girlfriend, Samantha, who is later revealed to be a biological male—a not-so-subtle suggestion of the challenges that biocultural complexity may present to traditional romantic-reproductive scripts. After the disruption, Nina and Dwayne leave and are pulled over by a Black police officer, who immediately orders Dwayne to step out of the car when he reaches for his pocket to get the license. The officer is acting as if Dwayne has a weapon, but Dwayne takes a ring box out of his pocket and hands it over to the officer who leans in to look at Nina. The viewer is invited to see that beautiful Nina and the good-looking officer are a better match. The officer tells Dwayne that Nina is "out of [his] league" and does not even give Dwayne a ticket—he takes pity on him and sends him off with "enjoy it while you can." When Dwayne gets back in the car, he notices that Nina is not there; she is riding away with the officer. Dwayne screams, "Nina!" and wakes up from his daydream. Nina is actually still in the car; he only imagined her choosing a Black man over him. Over the course of the film, Dwayne experiences similar daydreaming episodes that explore his fears, which reveal Walter Mitty–ish crises of self-confidence. This particular one implies his self-identification as Black (he expects a traffic stop to go wrong), but at the same time, it undermines this self-identification as it shows Dwayne feeling inadequate next to a Black man whose body matches his cultural identification and social expectations for a romantic pairing with Nina. The sequencing of scenes suggests that "something ain't right about

7. There are more layers of meaning in the scene, and some details may be found offensive by viewers, including implicit comparison of human and animal adoption and insensitive comments about rape.

Dwayne": he claims belonging in the culture by performing it, but he is also insecure about being perceived as not enough.

The encounter with the police officer is happening in Dwayne's imagination with the implication that the inadequacies are in his head. But there are also real reasons for his feeling uncertain about his identity and belonging. A few brief episodes show his interactions with the lager community that does not seem to accept him. A flashback to Dwayne getting lost in the supermarket suggests he is not being seen as part of his adoptive Black family when two Black security guards who found him act surprised at seeing Dolores, who comes to pick him up. Another scene, at the church, shows women judging Dolores for not giving a child to Harold and for not adopting a Black child. Instead of taking care of "our own," "she took care of an Oriental"—"Two!" The racism of these remarks is reiterated when one of the women openly says that the adoptees do not fit in: "Look at this poor baby. He needs to be with his own." Such thinking, which is often implied in cultural ideas about adoption, but which the comedy genre allows to stage openly, is counteracted with humor or mockery directed at the insensitive character in order to keep the viewer engaged when challenged to face some inconvenient truths about cultural perceptions of adoption. When church women turn to Dolores and Dwayne and fawn over him hypocritically, he pulls off a brooch that holds one of the women's outfits together and makes the half-naked woman run away, embarrassed. The same mechanism is used in the scene that shows adult Dwayne's real-world interaction with a Black man. An irate customer who is picketing the bank where Dwayne is a manager draws on the "middleman minority" stereotype to insult Dwayne, who is walking by. The film mocks his remark, "Chinese run this place," by showing that all people working in the bank are Black, except for Dwayne.

Over the course of the film, Dwayne's character development is built around acquiring confidence to pursue his relationship and marriage with Nina, which would make him more secure in his belonging in the Black culture and community. Unlike Julian from *Fakin',* Dwayne is not fully assimilated into the Black culture, and he eventually tries to gain some competency in the Vietnamese culture. But the plot still presents his identity as hinging on the need to make a choice between two cultures as he decides which reproductive future to pursue. His heterocoital origin is presented as disruptive to his adoptive belonging and his intended reproductive futurity when his insecurities intensify after the birth mother's arrival. Thanh estranges Dwayne from Nina by her presence and by deliberately manipulating him. Just when he proposes to Nina, Mai shows up and says she found the birth mother, stealing attention from the couple. When Nina is late to the welcome dinner for Thanh, Dwayne interprets it as a rejection. His fears provoke another daydreaming episode, in which the cat says to him, "Wake up man, you are short!" Thanh herself openly disapproves of Nina and tries to set up Dwayne with a Vietnamese woman. When she begins to criticize his involvement with Nina and the name given to him by the adoptive parents, Dwayne resists her attempts to control his identity and reproductive choices and draws a boundary between his origin and his adoptive identity. Yet, while Dwayne resists Thanh's provocations and tries to ignore her even when she moves in with him, he doubts himself and feels the need to figure out his connection to the birth family and culture.

It is significant that he finds an emotional outlet to deal with his past with Nina, not his birth mother or Mai. At a picnic with Nina, he cries and says he cannot remember what his birth father looked like. His resentment over being abandoned is directed at his birth mother because the birth father had to leave him and Mai at the embassy in order to go find the birth mother. His father never came back, but Dwayne seems to hold a grudge against the birth mother for disappearing and making the father look for her. The grudge seems to have held him back from taking interest in his birth culture and connecting with his birth mother. This intimate sharing not only strengthens Dwayne's bond with Nina but also makes him more open with Thanh. After the scene in the park, Dwayne accepts his birth name, Sap, and begins talking to his birth mother in Vietnamese. He tries to learn the language using tapes, and he shops at an Asian food market. The change represents Dwayne's acceptance of Thanh and Vietnamese culture as part of his identity, but the change is facilitated by a conversation with Nina—yet another suggestion of Dwayne's hybridity.

Thanh's aggressive involvement in Dwayne's life is a nod to the "birth mother shows up" scenario that is characteristic of adoption drama and a reversal of the trope of a silent or absent transnational birth mother. Thanh is not a grieving and unconditionally grateful birth mother who confirms the belonging of her children with the adoptive parents and remains on the sidelines. In fact, her character is acting out all possible threats to the adoptee and the adoptive family the figure of a birth mother may represent. She ignores Mai, who craves a close relationship with her and pursues closeness with Dwayne, who sees her as intrusive and controlling. One of the ways the film stages the influence of the birth mother on her children and the adoptive family is through her attempts to control their reproductive futurity. She tells Mai to start a family because she is "not getting any younger" and asks Mai to put her in touch with an old friend who has a daughter who could be a good match for Dwayne. The film couches often insensitive cultural stereotypes in comedy. For example, Thanh's aggressive matchmaking is mocked when she cluelessly asks Samantha, Michael's girlfriend, if she knows anyone like herself for Dwayne, who grunts disapprovingly at this suggestion. The film intends this scene, together with the following one, as pivotal to the overall theme about who is a good match for whom and why—a discussion that exposes the importance of biocultural consistency to maintaining socially legible categories of race and gender.

In the next scene, Dwayne and Michael are talking about the authenticity of Dwayne's Blackness together with the authenticity of Michael's desire for Samantha. Michael insists on his heterosexuality, against Dwayne's conviction that Michael must be gay if he is in a sexual relationship with a biological man. In this *M. Butterfly*-esque scenario, Michael claims that he is not gay and is not attracted to men. For Michael, Samantha's gender "depends [on] who you ask," and Samantha's gender identity defines her as a woman that he is attracted to. Dwayne, however, insists on Samantha being a "man" because she has a penis. This argument over biological bodily characteristic versus performance as a measure of who one is echoes the logic of figuring out who Dwayne is as an adoptee, meaning, what matters more: heterocoital genealogy and racialized body characteristics or his performance of cultural and racial identity that he experiences as his self? Is performance enough for others? While Michael seems to allow complexity in gender identifications, he uses Dwayne's rigid logic in naming who Dwayne is. He says, "And who are you? You sound like you are from the freaking hood. Dwayne, you are Vietnamese, for Christ's sake!" Dwayne responds, "Maaan, you trippin.'" Michael can engage with Samantha's performance as genuine since the performed identity confirms his own heterosexuality, but he cannot accept Dwayne's performance of Blackness as genuine. The comedic element is both Michael's and Dwayne's blindness to disrupted biocultural consistencies that they have to account for in pursuing the identities they want to claim. But they refuse to acknowledge their own and each other's complexity and continue to look at their situations in the light of traditional nature-culture correlations. The scene offers a snapshot of the process in which established cultural ideas insist on shaping shared reality, while the actions and internal states of characters signal that the intended reality is not shared. Cultural heterometaphors are not enough for understanding Michael's experience, and neither are heterocoital ones for Dwayne's.

Catfish opens up suggestive inconsistencies in biocultural scripts, but the resolution of the plot gravitates toward a reaffirmation of traditional kinship. The adoptees' relationships with Thanh are renegotiated to emotionally privilege the adoptive family, and Dwayne's reproductive future with Nina is confirmed and approved. Thanh's involvement in the reintegrated adoptive family is minimized with a simultaneous acknowledgment of her presence. She moves in with Mai and her husband, Vinh, but Mai acquires emotional distance from her birth mother in following the advice of Vinh, who says, "She does not care how you feel. You are not a child anymore. . . . You spent all this time looking for your mother. You found her. It's time to stop looking." Mai gets a mother she has been searching for after she understands that the Vietnamese mother may not be the (only) mother she needs. She finally lets Dolores in and allows her adoptive mother to comfort her. Dolores, who felt threatened by Thanh, reclaims her family by saying that they did a good job raising children and they should stop competing with "this woman." The concluding scene, of a family dinner, features the adoptive family together, Dwayne and Nina as a couple, and Thanh sitting by herself but acknowledged with a brief nod from Dolores. Michael and Samantha are bracketed out, even though their storyline is not abandoned. In a scene preceding the family dinner, we see their reconciliation after an argument. Sam is shown crying in their room, dressed like a man. After answering the knock on the door in a deep voice, which Michael responds to with a surprised "Samantha?," Sam shrieks, closes the door, and requests in a feminine voice, "Give me an hour." The sight of Samantha as a man "confirms" Dwayne's suspicions that Samantha's femininity is a performance and thus reactivates the viewers' commitment to a conventional biocultural script. But the situation with Samantha, as a foil for Dwayne's situation, underscores that such commitment relies on the acceptance of identity performance unsupported by the "right" biology as genuine, in order to maintain a culturally legible and socially acceptable relationship. Otherwise, openly expressed biocultural hybridity may not guarantee belonging and social cohesion, because it implies a divergent futurity and cannot assure a transfer of unhybridized culture. The outcome of such negotiations is reinstatement of heterocoital metaphors as *the* ways of thinking about family even in its non-heterocoital configurations. In order to give nonbiological kinship space to be the primary and only visible kinship that assures the transfer of the right culture, Samantha has to be accepted as a woman by Michael, who thinks of himself as a heterosexual man, and Dwayne has to be accepted (and accept himself) as Black enough to marry Nina. Both situations reveal to the viewer that such adjustments recast "natural" ways of belonging as cultural performances and modify the identities of all participants, not just the one who is portrayed as "adjusted." They show that heterocoital scripts can organize, and insist on organizing, identities and belonging even in the absence of heterocoital reproduction, even as they become simulacra untethered from lived experiences.

All adoption narratives are working out a stance on non-heterocoital family and biocultural hybridity, but while other genres may lead to more conservative outcomes, and while even comedies may eventually wrap up all subversive storylines in a reinstatement of the status quo, comedy allows the viewer to go into the realm where hybridity is lived, at least as a possibility. Celestino Deleyto describes a typical narrative arc of a romantic (Shakespearean) comedy as going away from familiar society into an unfamiliar one, "in the course of which . . . the characters learn something about themselves . . . and, armed with the strengths conferred by this new identity, they return to take up their rightful positions in their social group" (31). At the same time, King observes that comedy may work to "bring together . . . characters from very different backgrounds," and, in fact, it troubles the homogeneity of social groups, which is maintained through kinship practices (53). Deleyto himself states that even though romantic comedy "articulates ideological discourses in the field of affective and sexual relationships," it does not "tell us what to think or how to behave" and suggests looking at the middle of a comedic narrative as "its main discursive space" (18, 28–29). In other words, the narrative middle of a romantic comedy may expose a broader range of affective, sexual, and reproductive expressions than a happy ending would allow.

Heterocoital transgressions of adoptive comedy offer a Bakhtinian carnivalesque experience, a "departure[e] from the conventions of everyday life" (King 8), where viewers can "act out fantasies" (Horton and Rapf 3). In other words, while horror presents a transgression as a threat, and in melodrama it offers a reason for tragedy, comedy shows what we might *gain* from transgressing the boundaries of the heterocoital order. By putting the possibilities on the table, comedy shows its viewers a revised social order as it immerses them into a socially suspect structure of feeling that nevertheless may be experienced as desirable and pleasurable. The threat inherent in the transgression is modulated by humor and laughter. Such possibilities are often located in the secondary plotlines and characters that resist the comedy ending's drive toward restoring the order. In this way, the queerness of the nontraditional kinship situation may be displaced onto and not fully resolved in the secondary characters' storylines. In *Catfish,* for instance, the profusion of minor storylines and characters, which is often read by critics as a drawback of the script and the director's failure to contain the narrative, may very well be a running commentary on culturally acceptable kinship narratives that the film puts in question.

While queered futurities are not heterocoitally reproduced and are relegated to the margins, they are not done away with. Neither are they presented as threats similar to the horror genre trope of the "hidden spring." They remain ridiculously untenable, unlikely, and unreproducible, yet they remain a possibility. In this way, adoption comedies follow the logic of the genre as described by King, who sees in it two conflicting undercurrents and thinks that comedy can be "both subversive, questioning the norms from which it departs, and affirmative, reconfirming that which it recognizes through the act of departure; or a mixture of the two" (8). Such mixture may lead to narratives that affirm heterocoital reproduction and kinship within the larger narrative arc but subvert it at the level of individual characters (even the main ones) and secondary storylines. At the same time, more than in other genres, the ethos of comedy allows for explorations of variety and nuance in subject positions of nontraditional kinship participants, as comedy more rigorously resists the production of a "single story." For example, Dwayne and Mai follow quite different paths as adult adopted persons, and Julian chooses not to engage with the common cultural expectation to connect to his origin.

Raising Arizona is an adoption rom-com that plays with such conventions and "clears the field" for alternative imaginings of kinship by exposing both the nuclear heterocoital and adoptive families as unrealistic ideals. The film conspicuously extends the romance plot into its telos—heterocoital reproduction—and portrays any kind of family that is a biological nuclear family or an imitation of it as dysfunctional and not quite reproducing the cultural values associated with this traditional form of kinship. In *Raising Arizona,* the need of a romantic couple to have a baby is portrayed as a condition for the stability of their romantic union. The premise of the plot is the inability of the newlyweds Hi (a small-time crook) and Edwina (a police officer) to start a family because of Ed's (Holly Hunter) infertility and Hi's (Nicolas Cage) criminal record making them ineligible for adopting a child. The couple decides to kidnap a baby of Nathan and Florence Arizona (Trey Wilson and Lynne Kitei), who have just had quintuplets and publicly admitted that "it's more than [they] can handle." Critics often read the film as two romantic comedies by separating what happens before and after the credits. Jeffrey Melton, for instance, reads the film through the rom com's "how will they get together?" (8) trope and sees the first eleven minutes, which are a condensed representation of Ed and Hi's romance and how it ends up in marriage, as "a romantic comedy in microcosm" (5). For Melton, the opening sequence culminates in the sunset scene—Hi and Ed in lawn chairs enjoying the view—which provides an "image of domestic tranquility" and "a pleasant closing to the whirlwind romance," which "points toward an idyllic future wholly compatible with American mythology" (6). Hi and Ed's pursuit of parenthood is understood here as a claim to middle-class status and an opportunity for social rehabilitation for Hi. The nuclear family institution, in other words, is positioned as a guarantor of social order and upward mobility, and its reproductive potential is assumed. But the last thing that happens before the film's title burns onto the screen is the couple's decision to kidnap a child to "complete" their family because they cannot reproduce heterocoitally. They are shown driving into the sunset having secured a ladder to the roof of their car.

In the course of the film, Hi and Ed discover that even one child is more than *they* can handle, and they make a responsible decision to return the stolen baby to the Arizonas. On its face, the plot of the film seems to end in an affirmation of the structure of a family that assures the child's interests: a heterocoital nuclear family with a social class standing that signals responsible parenting and enough means to provide good childcare. But the Arizonas are not, in fact, a traditional heterocoital family. Florence "had been taking fertility pills" to get pregnant, and her giving birth to quintuplets is beyond normative cultural expectations for human reproduction. Nathan Arizona does not come across as a responsible father when he cannot remember the names of his children and callously uses Nathan Jr.'s kidnapping as an opportunity to promote his business on TV. The adoption plot built around Hi and Ed fails to sustain values associated with the traditional heterocoital family that adoptive families are supposed to imitate. Hi and Ed's storyline is actually a reversal of the typical adoption scenario in which adoptive parents are more responsible and financially secure than birth parents. Other potential caregivers of Nathan Jr. are no better. Gale and Evelle, Hi's escaped prisonmates, steal the baby to get the bounty money. Hi's morally suspect boss, Glen, tries to blackmail Hi into giving him Nathan Jr., so Glen's wife, Dot, can enjoy another baby while he is still "cuddly." Dot and Glen can barely manage the children they already have, though. Leonard Smalls, the biker bounty hunter, is hunting the baby to either get an increased reward from Nathan Arizona or sell the baby on the black market. The baby is passed among caregivers who can hardly provide safety and competent care, and during all the escapades, Nathan Jr. miraculously remains unharmed even though his life is repeatedly endangered. Childcare "success" ascribed to the middle-class nuclear family begins to look just as accidental as the "success" of the various crooks who have had the child in their care, while Florence Arizona, his upstanding mother, could not assure the baby's safety. Given that, the seemingly happy ending that returns the baby to his biological parents still leaves the viewer with mixed feelings about the cultural tendency to value the middle-class nuclear family model over other forms of childcare and kinship.

As a continuous roast of this traditional family, *Raising Arizona* puts the social and monetary value of the baby out in the open—a departure from the view of the child-parent bond as built on emotional attachment, with the financial and social underpinnings of reproduction carefully concealed behind unconditional parental love. Talking about his "informal adoption," Hi says, "It's like when I was robbing convenience stores." He makes a point of having taken the best baby. Gale and Evelle get attached to Nathan Jr. and consider the option of getting the reward against starting their own "family" with him—a clear separation of the child's monetary and emotional values. The storyline that connects Hi and Leonard Smalls and suggests that the bounty hunter is Hi's alter ego[8] links Hi's own orphanhood to Smalls's story. The bounty hunter, who has a "mother didn't love me" tattoo and carries a pair of bronzed baby shoes on his belt as a reminder of his childhood, hints that he himself brought about thirty thousand dollars on the baby black market. The film ups the ante in its running joke about traditional family as a sham by comparing the prison to a form of kinship. During a counseling session in prison, the counselor tells Hi that men his age get married and raise a family; Hi tries to object, "Well, actually . . . ," but the counselor interrupts: "They wouldn't accept prison as a substitute," suggesting that Hi may be looking at the prison as such. And indeed, when Hi is walking into the prison the second time, he says that it feels almost like a "homecoming," because faces, smells, and voices are familiar to him. The ending of the film solidifies the idea that a happy nuclear family is a myth. It is shot in soft focus that signals an unrealistic dream and suggests that Ed and Hi may not stay together after returning the baby. Hi tries to wish a reproductive future into existence by fantasizing about getting old with Ed and being surrounded by their children and grandchildren. The contrast with the overall aesthetic of the film even more directly insinuates that the heterocoital nuclear family may not be a "natural" human state but, rather, a dream, a cultural construct accessible only to those with the means to perform it. *Raising Arizona* thus exposes the heterocoital family together with its imitations as failing to live up to the cultural ideal and invites audiences to accept this, with laughter. This exposure of heterocoital family performativity, however, does not decenter it as an organizing principle of Western culture and human identity. The outcome of *Raising Arizona* is an acceptance of the heterocoital family dream, akin to the cultural acceptance of the American dream that survives as a powerful culture-structuring metaphor, all its critiques notwithstanding. The power of this myth manifests itself when Nathan Arizona's ART family is imagined as heterocoital due to the biological link between children and both parents and its "heterocoital enough" method of assisted reproduction (fertility pills).

8. See Sanders for a more detailed discussion of this connection.

Cinematic narratives that represent more radical methods of assisted reproduction have to work harder to reconcile them with the cultural demand to preserve the heterocoital family as the norm. At the same time, they show more clearly what is at stake in its preservation. For example, sperm donation comedies negotiate deep cultural anxieties about challenges to heterocoital reproduction posed by sperm "alienation" in this process (O'Brien 1989, 97). Even though this method of assisted reproduction is widely accepted and practiced, the previous chapter's analysis of ART horror films has shown that the patriarchy may be unsettled by it, especially if the alienation is portrayed as a loss of control over sperm's potential uses at the hands of the monstrous feminine hell-bent on revising "the natural order of things." Comedies approach the subject with what seems like a lighter touch and aim to manage through laughter what Mary O'Brien recognizes as the patriarchy's anxiety over the fact that "men are . . . separated *materially* from both nature and biological continuity by the alienation of the male seed in copulation" (97). O'Brien's Marxist analysis of the differences in male and female reproductive consciousness can help understanding of the negotiations around assisted reproductive technologies represented in ART comedies. While her ideas have been subjected to critique due to inattention to intersectional identities, her analysis of differences in male and female reproductive experiences as the basis for the patriarchal culture may lead to some explanations of the persistence of the heterocoital order. O'Brien argues that experiences of gestation and labor, attributed to those with female bodies, provide a sense of continuity and an organic connection to the future of the species, even if the potential for birth remains just culturally presumed and not actually fulfilled in cases of individual women.[9] In other words, O'Brien theorizes female group consciousness as a sense of uninterrupted continuity of humanity through time, grounded in the way natural pregnancy and birth are experienced by women. "What is really 'natural' for men is discontinuity," O'Brien writes as she points

9. Carla Lam responds to critiques of Mary O'Brien's concept of reproductive consciousness as limited to only those who can experience gestation and birth by explaining that the gendered consciousnesses O'Brien describes need to be understood as akin to Jungian collective consciousness that informs cultural schemas for organizing individual psyches and social structures. She writes: "Women's reproduction gives rise to particular gendered subjectivity—men's and women's reproductive consciousnesses—regardless of whether individual women reproduce or individual men nurture and care for babies and children. For example, we do not have to use IVF to be affected by the technomaterial and cultural disembodiment of reproduction that follows from the new reproductive technologies" (Lam 83). Also see Annette Burfoot for a response to critiques of O'Brien based on her inattention to "race, global positioning, sexual orientation, and . . . class" (179) in her Marxist analysis of "human procreation" as "the ultimate materialist basis for social relationships" (175). Burfoot claims that the concept of "reproductive consciousness" can still "guide political responses to contemporary problems raised by new reproductive technologies" (175).

out that men's participation in reproduction ends at coitus, which may not be enough to experience a connection to the child—the link to futurity (137). She explains that the need to create a sense of continuity and viable future is mediated by the male reproductive consciousness through creation of the patriarchal culture that can be then transmitted through generations as a way of assuring futurity. To provide a sense of permanency to culture, it needs to be hitched to the recursive biological process of reproduction, and biocultural kinship seems to be the concept that achieves that. O'Brien attributes the emergence of patriarchy to the discovery of known paternity—a discovery that establishes the need and a place for a man within the continuity of biological reproduction. But this place is precarious: until recently it has not been possible to know which particular man's sperm was involved in reproducing a child without knowing which man was present at copulation and if he was the only one who had access to a particular woman. In response to this precarity and as a way to ground men's control over the reproductive resources, the patriarchy relies on institutions such as monogamy and heterocoital family that help establish known paternity—the root cause of the imperative to know one's biological parents as a condition for "complete" selfhood. These institutions and ideas tie the "abstract idea" of "paternity" to the concrete act of copulation of "one particular man" with a woman (O'Brien 1989, 29–30). Cultural imperative to know one's origin can then be understood as the imperative to establish paternity as a condition of the universal human origin.[10]

Known paternity certifies male presence at conception as an ingredient in the process of continuing life and perpetuating the human species, and it serves as the basis for men's appropriation of children, which O'Brien characterizes as "a culturally structured *right* to appropriate women's reproductive labor and to redefine their own exclusion from species continuity as freedom" (15).[11] O'Brien's Marxist approach treats reproduction as production and a

10. Adoption narratives show that, in the absence of knowledge about biological parents, the need to search for the mother may take precedence over searching for a father, which points to the perceived primacy of biological continuity along the mother-child line of gestation and labor. The presence of a man at conception is assumed. The search for a specific father may often reveal preoccupations with legitimacy and social recognition, or it can be carried out if it is impossible to find the mother.

11. O'Brien's conceptualization of the specifics of male and female reproductive consciousnesses provides an interesting angle for possible analyses of search narratives, both dealing with adoption and with ART, since it hints at the reasons for cultural insistence on the need to know one's heterocoital origin and the ways through which this information is sought and becomes known. For example, adoption searches are often for mothers (might it really be about the gestation and labor aspect of origin?), while in ART situations where the mother is known, the search for the father comes to the fore. Narratives of surrogacy may offer yet another scenario to think through. Complexities of such analysis, however, are beyond the scope of this book.

basis for a sociopolitical structure. In other words, the ways in which reproduction is organized—alienated males usurping and manipulating female reproductive power—assure that "the abstracted father is reintegrated through the concreteness of patriarchal culture" (15). Given the importance of known paternity as an organizing principle for the patriarchy, heterocoitus, as a pillar of it, appears to be even more important than heterosexuality. Compulsory heterosexuality serves to assure heterocoital reproduction, but heterocoitus is the point of entrance of the man into species continuity and conceivable futurity. The need to freeze this point in time and to possess knowledge of it informs patriarchal imagination, and we can see this in cinematic narratives focused on male roles in assisted reproduction.

Specifically, romantic comedies can manage this need through the already familiar reimagining of nontraditional reproduction along heterocoital lines. In "Something Else Besides a Father," an examination of romantic comedies that focus on assisted reproduction via sperm donation, Jennifer Maher claims that while such films challenge the "primacy of the heterosexual couple" in reproduction by positing the possibility of reproduction outside heterosexuality, their endings still insist on the "'socially foundational status of the male-female couple'" (864).[12] Maher observes in these comedies a "cultural anxiety evinced by the figure of the unattached mother" (854) and shows that, while they assert, to a degree, female bodily autonomy and freedom to reproduce outside of the heterosexual coupling, in the end, the "unattached mother" is brought back into the heteronormative fold through the logic of the "'natural' romance of the patriarchal family" (855). In the films Maher considers, women who resort to sperm donor assistance end up in heterosexual relationships, often with the very donor who provided the sperm. In other words, heterocoital configuration of human reproduction is reestablished, even if it is post-factum.

More interesting effects of ARTs on culture can be observed, however, if we look at the films that feature men as the main characters of the reproduction plot. While there may be several variations of this type of ART comedy, this chapter will consider *Delivery Man* (2013) and *Junior* (1994) as representative, respectively, of one of the most popular themes—the prolific sperm donor—and one of the most transgressive subjects in reproduction—the pregnant man. The prolific-sperm-donor plot was extensively used in comedy around the 2010s. *Delivery Man* is a remake of *Starbuck* (2011); other films and TV shows with the similar theme are *Super Dad* (2015), *Seed* (2013), *Vicky*

12. She analyzes comedies like *Baby Mama* (2008), *The Switch* (2010), and *The Back-Up Plan* (2010).

Donor (2012), and *Fonzy* (2013). Unlike the horror genre that amplifies anxieties over sperm alienation and its subsequent uncontrolled and "unnatural" use, the comedy treats the possibility of sperm-donor fatherhood as an intriguing possibility for the patriarchy and as a way to amplify its power. *Junior* and other films, like *Rabbit Test* (1978) and *Paternity Leave* (2015), that explore the possibility of male pregnancy are less common, perhaps, because they push the envelope a bit further. They explore social consequences of male pregnancy that could upend the heterocoital order in more profound ways. This makes them fascinating objects of analysis that can uncover the intricate representational footwork such narratives do to negotiate integration of nontraditional reproduction into patriarchal, heterocoital cultures.

In *Delivery Man,* David Wozniak (Vince Vaughn), who has donated his sperm anonymously over 600 times, is threatened by a lawsuit initiated by 142 out of 533 of his biological children, who want to know his identity. At the same time, he finds out that his girlfriend, Emma (Cobie Smulders), is pregnant with his child but is hesitating to acknowledge him as a father because he is irresponsible and immature. The plot of the film is bringing this conflict to a resolution by showing David "grow up" as he is making himself present in the lives of his biological children at the same time as he is trying to be a reliable partner for his girlfriend and a father to their child. In *Delivery Man* thus the sperm donor's biological fatherhood of 533 children is normalized by his performance of social fatherhood in relation to both his heterocoital child and the children begotten by sperm donation. This representation shores up the cultural importance of social fatherhood and positions David as restored to traditional heterocoital patriarchal fatherhood, with the biological and the social aspects of it seamlessly connected. At the same time, his reproductive prowess is "scaled up"—the fact of multiple offspring is treated by the film as an exciting new possibility for masculinity. The echoes of Dr. Hindle's megalomaniacal aspirations from *False Positive* are hard to ignore here, but the comedy genre puts a positive spin on what otherwise might look like a nightmare.

Junior works through the unlikely scenario of the pregnant man by imagining the scientific-experiment-gone-rogue scenario as leading to a successful birth that creates a nuclear family in the end. Fertility researcher Alex Hesse (Arnold Schwarzenegger) and fertility practitioner Larry Arbogast (Danny DeVito) decide to prove the efficacy of an anti-miscarriage drug by testing it on Alex after the FDA denies permission to use it on female human subjects. Larry implants a fertilized human egg (stolen from fellow researcher Diana Reddin, played by Emma Thompson) in Alex's abdomen, hoping to end the experiment in three months after they acquire the data needed to sell it to a big pharma company. But pregnancy changes Alex, and he wants to carry the child to term. Hijinks ensue as Alex is trying to conceal the changes in his body and character, while the stakes are raised after Diana finds out the truth and the research university that originally sponsored Alex and Larry's experiment decides to appropriate its outcome. In the end, Alex and Diana get romantically involved and are shown bringing up the successfully delivered child together.

While *Junior* toys with a more radical revision of reproduction than *Delivery Man* by decentering women's central role in gestation and labor and extending men's participation in the reproductive process beyond sperm alienation, the outcome of this revision is less radical than the one offered by *Delivery Man. Delivery Man* keeps women out of the picture almost entirely as it insists on normalization of the sperm-donor's multiple paternity. Its idea of reproduction "without" women makes this comedy a rather unsettling premonition of the patriarchy's possible response to ARTs and speaks to the concern some feminist scholars of ARTs have articulated as the patriarchal tendency to imagine women's role in reproduction as body parts (wombs, ovaries) or social functions (wife, mother), or both, rather than self-determining subjects.[13] And while representations of such tendencies in the horror genre produce due anxieties, comedy minimizes them by sentimentalizing social fatherhood and minimizing traditional expressions of masculinity in the sperm donor. David is often described as an "affable underachiever" ("*Delivery Man*," *IMDB* synopsis) or "amiable slacker" ("*Delivery Man*," *Rotten Tomatoes* synopsis) by film critics who see *Delivery Man* as a "heartwarming comedy" ("*The Delivery Man*," *Amazon* description)—a far cry from the evil narcissist of the horror genre who wants to take over the world with his progeny. Even as he comes into his own and "appropriate[s]" (O'Brien 1989, 15) children conceived with his sperm, he remains "a good man" loved by everybody. Such redefinitions of masculinity may be, according to Maher, a "strategy of masculine representation that can . . . rehabilitat[e] [men] in order to not appear obsolete in this new (post-feminist) world of sperm for sale" (858). But they also announce troubling developments that emerge when heterocoital cultures adjust to the new reproductive landscape aiming to preserve structures that facilitate appropriation of female reproductive power.

Junior explores and exposes patriarchal uses of gendered reproductive roles as it works toward an (often misguided) vision of reproductive equity by stitching together the differences between male and female reproductive consciousnesses as theorized by O'Brien. *Junior* aims to rehabilitate masculinity

13. See a more detailed discussion of this scholarship in the conclusion.

by revising male reproductive consciousness through showing the effects of gestation on a pregnant man. Alex undergoes physical changes induced by the pregnancy and female hormones he is taking to sustain it, and the progression of these changes is portrayed as his introduction to female reproductive experiences. Obsessively organized and pedantic at first, Alex gradually relaxes and learns to appreciate life's pleasures and emotional experiences as his connection to the growing fetus develops into what culture would recognize as the mother-child bond and O'Brien would call a material connection to "biological [species] continuity" (97). Given the genre, though, these transformations are presented as humorous drag punctuated with quips by Larry that bring Alex back to patriarchal reality and remind him of what masculinity is supposed to be. In the end, masculinity, or male reproductive consciousness, is not revised to a radical extent. At most, it is reversed without revision for a while as Alex is shown becoming a stereotypical woman. At best, he is becoming the "sensitive man" of the rom com—a revision that does not profoundly challenge the gendered structures of patriarchy.

Nevertheless, representation of Alex's transformation provokes reflection on the significance of the gestation process as a stage in reproduction. In *Junior,* it is simultaneously presented as not "natural" to women and thus as available to men, yet it is also renaturalized and reassigned to women by suggesting that to be capable of carrying a baby, one must become what is recognized culturally, and to a degree biologically, as a woman. The film opens with a dream sequence that shows Alex in a library doing research. He hears a baby crying, and the camera follows his POV as he is moving around until he sees a baby on top of the circulation desk. Alex looks lost; he tries to attract attention by saying, "Hello! There is a baby here! There *must* be a mother! Hello!?" (emphasis mine). No one answers him, so he decides to put down the books and pick up the baby. The baby pees itself, to Alex's dismay, and he cries for help. As he is walking around trying to find someone who can take the baby off his hands, he sees rows of armchairs, each one holding two fussing babies. At this moment, Alex wakes up, terrified and then relieved. He starts doing abdominal crunches as if trying to reconfirm that a man's body is for working out, not for babies. The next scene shows him at his work at a research university, explaining to his students that a "miscarriage-prone female's reproductive system is merely an extension of the body's *natural and necessary* instincts to reject foreign matter. . . . The body mistakenly identifies the embryo as an unwanted foreign substance and creates antibodies to fight and reject it" (emphasis mine). A suggestion is made here that carrying a child may not be natural for anyone. In fact, embryo rejection is recognized as the female body's natural resistance to "foreign matter," even though this response is labeled as mistaken and the "natural and necessary instinct" is limited to women who experience miscarriages. On the one hand, Alex sounds like he is naturalizing miscarriages as opposed to seeing them as a disability. On the other, by calling the embryo a "foreign substance," his speech is laying the groundwork for the idea that a man's body may be able to deal with this foreign substance if helped with the right drugs, just like the drugs that they are developing with Larry to help women's bodies carry a child to term.

Through Alex's personal negotiation of his role as a very masculine scientist in control of an experiment vis-à-vis his role as a gestating father who is losing his sense of the gender binary, *Junior* is playing with potential revisions of reproductive discourses. Alex is persuaded to experiment on himself by Larry, who appeals to Alex's scientific ambition and narcissism by comparing the impact of this experiment to Edward Jenner injecting himself with smallpox to test the vaccine. Larry urges Alex to "claim [his] place in the pantheon," and even though Alex knows that he is being manipulated, he agrees. His sense of the masculine reproductive role's importance is boosted by Larry, who praises Alex's sperm, contained in a jar: "Way to go!"; "Terrific motility"; "Excellent count"; "Strong swimmers"; "Big load." In contrast to ART films' scenes of implantation that involve women, which are typically suggestive of some "miracle of life" taking place, Alex's implantation scene looks rather like a biohacking experiment. Alex's face is either wincing or unemotional. The focus is not on him or Larry but on the ultrasound machine screen and the IVF needle. The lab is dark. Alex is still dressed in his black suit pants, not a hospital gown, and his naked torso underscores his masculine physique. Him and Larry are shown as research partners making decisions together about where to implant the embryo. When the camera's focus shifts to Larry's finger depressing the plunger that sends the embryo into Alex's abdominal cavity, there is no implied comparison to a sexual reproductive act. There is no hint that "impregnation" has any heterosexual overtones. However, the next scene is a dream sequence that shows Alex in a brightly lit hospital room filled with flowers and wearing a hospital gown. The scene begins with a close-up of Alex's relaxed face. He looks like he is just waking up. A sexy nurse brings him a baby that (the horror!) has Alex's own grown-up-looking face.[14] The baby says, "Mama," and Alex looks around trying to figure out where the baby's mama is. It dawns on him that he is the mama, and he wakes up in horror.

---

14. This brief horrific glimpse of "men reproducing themselves" as the outcome of assisted reproduction is shut down right away in this sequence by designating Alex very swiftly as a "mama." A more recent TV show, *Foundation,* analyzed in the conclusion of this book, develops this idea with less restraint and offers a vision of the patriarchy empowered through recursive male self-reproduction.

He does not wake up in the lab, though. He is now in a femininely appointed room (Larry's ex-wife's) in Larry's house, where he is supposed to stay for the duration of the experiment. The setting and the lack of memory about transfer to Larry's house from the lab are the first inklings of his losing control over his freedom and body. The erosion of his role as Larry's research partner is also suggested by showing Larry's increasing treatment of Alex as one of his fertility patients.

While Alex behaves as a scientist in control of the experiment for a while after the implantation, eventually, as he and Larry have to raise the dose of his hormone supplements to prevent a miscarriage, his emotional expression begins to resemble that of the stereotypical "pregnant woman" with mood swings. He suffers from morning sickness, his nipples become too sensitive, he has cramps that he can hardly handle, and he confesses that he "feel[s] . . . humiliated." Larry meets his complaints with "It's perfectly normal," which shows that he begins to see Alex as one of his female patients, for whom such symptoms of pregnancy would be within the norm. By talking about his symptoms as caused by uncontrolled weight gain, Alex manages to get some empathetic support from Diana, who commiserates with him by sharing that women's bodies are out of control from puberty to menopause. Alex rejects such loss of control and says, "I never wanted to be a woman," but the film insists that someone who carries a child must become one.

As his pregnancy progresses, Alex is shown reading maternity magazines, eating too much food and in weird combinations, and crying while watching weddings on TV. A lot of the humor in the film is created through dialogue between Larry and Alex in which they behave as stereotypical husband and wife. In one of the scenes, Alex shares that he is not feeling like himself, and his request to be seen and heard by Larry is followed by an exchange that a busy husband and a jealous housewife could have, one about Larry going to a convention to meet potential drug-buyers and Alex pleading to join him because he has been feeling "pregnant and alone." Larry reminds Alex that he is not "*pregnant* pregnant" and that it is just an experiment. Alex seems to accept this, yet when Larry finally invites him to come along to the convention, Alex says, "but I have nothing to wear!" Alex's change is emphasized at the convention event as well, as he is enjoying massages and naps at the spa instead of attending presentations, tries different food, socializes with people, and dances with Diana. He is shown becoming more emotionally open, which may signal a development of "a different political understanding and relation to the natural and social realms" brought on by an experience of a "natural continuity that is sensed" now by Alex (Brodribb 260). But the logic of humor constantly signals that Alex is culturally perceived as turning into a woman, not becoming a new kind of man, and that he needs to be brought back to the reality of being a man. Even though Larry is a character who contributes to Alex's feminine transformation by treating him as a pregnant woman, he is also the "voice of reason" that reminds Alex to "get a grip" and remember what they are doing. At the same time, he excludes Alex from the business side of their project and relegates the labor of "data production" to him, effectively reinforcing a gendered labor division in their relationship. Still, it is understood that they both will benefit equitably from selling their research to drug companies. Such constant equivocation creates humorous situations by taking the narrative toward, and back from the brink of, imagining a world where a different relationship to reproduction turns men into women. The lack of significant change, however, exposes limited imaginative space for conceptualizing reproductive labor outside of the patriarchal gendered framework.

When transformed Alex makes a choice against Larry's wishes to take the baby to term because he now feels the "absolute joy and connection that carrying your baby brings" and is ready to "protect and nurture that miracle with everything [he's] got," he is confronted by Larry, who does not sugarcoat patriarchal truths this time. Larry admonishes, "You are a guy, Alex! This is totally against the natural order. Guys do not have babies. We leave it to the women. That's part of the beauty of being a guy. Didn't your father ever have this talk with you?" The conflation of the natural (or, rather, drug-induced) connection a pregnant man feels with a baby and life in general with renaturalized patriarchal ideas in this exchange is a blatant display of the patriarchal order at a loss when confronted with a different kind of reproductive consciousness, now empowered by its attachment to masculinity. Larry's mentioning of the "talk," which implies intergenerational knowledge transmission, points to the importance of the patriarchal culture transfer that Alex is messing up. The film deals with the potential challenges posed to the patriarchy by the revised male reproductive consciousness by reinscribing the gender binary and portraying any revisions as distinctively female: Alex is turning into a woman. His femaleness is enhanced to a grotesque degree when he goes into hiding in a home for expectant mothers disguised as a woman. To fulfill his desire of having a child, he must become a woman socially and accept seemingly benevolent limitations to his freedom and social power. The conflation of gender and sex as well as biological and social aspects of womanhood in this plot move aims to stitch biology and gender back together after a disruption of this seemingly natural connection. And the erosion of Alex's patriarchal masculinity as a result of his revised reproductive role is halted by presenting Alex's experience as being in the service of creating a heterocoital, heterosexual, nuclear family.

Even though he is consistently emasculated, Alex's heterosexuality is maintained throughout the film via his growing romantic involvement with Diana. The conventional rom com plot takes them from their meet-cute (Alex stops a cryogenic tank with Diana on top of it from rolling into a wall); to a Prince-Charming-like dancing scene at the convention; to Diana's confession that she feels a strangely strong connection to him and gets "pangs of concern for [his] well-being" followed by their first sexual contact; to Diana's eventual acceptance of the situation that ultimately leads to her and Alex becoming a family where each of the parents has borne a child. To keep the story of the unnatural conception on the heterocoital track, the film applies reverse logic to the reproduction process. As his attraction to Diana grows, Alex begins to believe that it was all a divine plan for him to get a baby and find a suitable woman. Just when he shares these thoughts with Larry, it comes out that the egg Larry stole was, in fact, Diana's, and the vial holding it was labeled "Junior"—exactly the name Alex gave his unborn baby. The "divine plan" to bring the heterocoital family together postconception is certified with a heterocoital act when Diana, who visits Alex in the home for expectant mothers, says, "Call me old-fashioned, but I'll be damned if I'm having a child with a man I never slept with," which she proceeds to do. The final scene of the film shows Alex and Diana together with Larry and his now former ex-wife, having a day at the beach with their children. Diana is pregnant, presumably heterocoitally, and thus the order is restored. Larry's family also looks indistinguishable from a heterocoital one, even though his wife was impregnated by the rock group Aerosmith's personal trainer. In other words, all the evidence of non-heterocoital and paternity-switching transgressions has been successfully covered, and it does not appear to matter what actual reproductive processes brought Alex's and Larry's firstborns into the world. The last shots of the film show everyone trying to convince Larry to bear a child and him vehemently refusing and running away. Ultimately, the film shows male pregnancy as possible but nonreproducible. The structure of reproductive labor that underlies the patriarchy remains unchanged: the heterocoital family remains; women continue reproductive labor, now made more efficient by the drug Larry and Alex developed; and men retain the power to appropriate the outcomes of this labor.

The imaginative potential for exploring revisions of cultural ideas about reproduction remains controlled in *Junior* by traditional ways of thinking. Still, it does introduce the uncertainty about the ownership and belonging of the ART-conceived child, even though it is obscured by the film's ending. Throughout the film, all parties to this nontraditional reproduction argue over whose baby Junior is and what the grounds for claiming the baby are, often

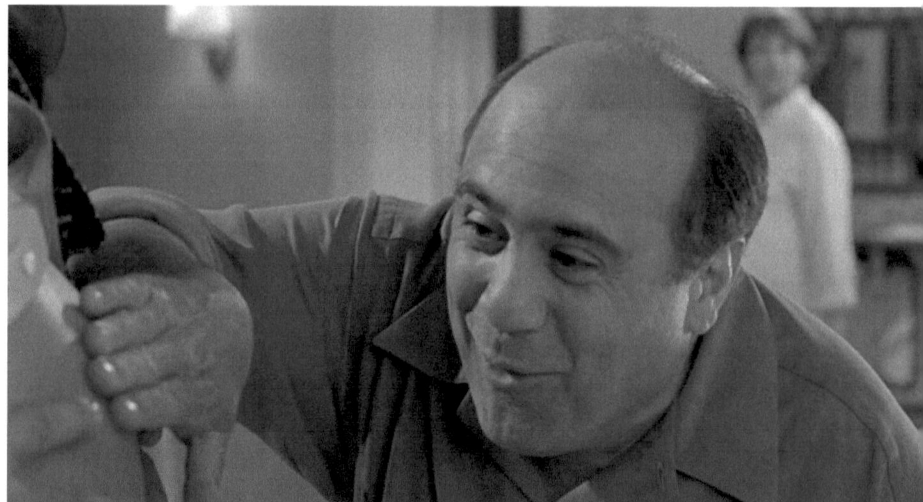

FIGURE 3.2. Larry fawning over Alex's pregnant belly in *Junior*. Universal Pictures, 1994.

to a comedic effect since the heterocoital ways of thinking do not map onto the situation at hand. "I'm gonna be a mama too," Alex says to Larry's pregnant ex-wife when she walks in on them fawning over Junior kicking Alex's belly (see figure 3.2). She reacts to the "exciting" news by fainting. When Alex and Larry talk about the possibility of birth, Alex is reassured when Larry says that he hopes everything is going to be all right because "it's [his] baby too." When Diana comes to visit Alex at the home for expectant mothers to negotiate their parental roles, she says that she still thinks it is "monumentally unfair" that he has done this. Alex reacts by leaning into the "unwanted pregnancy" cliché and says that he can "take the full responsibility for the baby," but Diana means something else. She responds, "Wait! Can we just get one thing straight here? This is my baby too. Don't you ever forget that. . . . I'm the mother. You're the father." She deals with her lack of physical connection to the child by reclaiming the social role of the mother. To Diana's doubt about her uncertain maternity—"And I thought that I would be . . ."—Alex responds with a firm "You are!" that stops this line of questions. The normalization of the situation is solidified by their immediate agreement to "do this together," which follows the heterocoital script and connects "normal upbringing" to gendered social roles (mother-female; father-male) and the family's purpose ("security," "safe home life"), even though the biology of the reproductive process is different.

More sinister negotiations of the child's ownership happen when the more overt representatives of the patriarchy—Larry and the head of the research lab—appear on the scene. The lack of heterocoital clarity about whose baby it is reveals that patriarchal power may work to appropriate non-heterocoital reproductive labor by reimagining it as technological production. While Larry is a more affable representative of the patriarchy who is often shown in a humorous key, his desire to help women have babies is clearly connected to his need to turn a profit. To him, the baby is both a sentimental object and a potential cash cow that will draw investments from drug companies. As a blunt voice of the patriarchy, he is telling Diana what she is afraid to hear. When they both arrive to the expectant mothers' home to help Alex, who begins to experience "contractions," Diana and Larry squabble over their roles in this situation. Larry is obviously annoyed by Diana's involvement and asks, "what are you doing here?" Diana responds, "It's my baby, not yours!" "I put it in there," quips Larry. "My egg," says Diana resorting to what she perceives as the ultimate biogenetic argument. Larry's comeback weaponizes the cultural cliché of a deadbeat father to deliver an uncomfortable truth: "Just because your egg's in some guy doesn't make you a mother." He confirms Diana's fears of disempowerment due to a techno-social change that makes "what was once certain, maternity, . . . uncertain" (Brodribb, ctd. in Burfoot 184). This exchange presents a vivid counterargument to the idea that reproductive freedom facilitates women's control over their bodies, gametes included. During the delivery, Larry keeps Diana out of the operation room. She can assist Larry's pregnant ex-wife, who goes into labor on the waiting room floor, but she cannot help with or be present at the delivery of her own child just a few feet away. The scene privileges male technologically assisted delivery and leaves a pregnant woman to deal with her natural birth with the help of another woman, who is not a doctor. This may look like a welcome acknowledgment of a woman's control over her body and a celebration of female mutual care outside of institutionalized reproductive medicine, except Larry's ex-wife wants "Drugs!" while she is second in line and all attention is consumed by Alex. Interestingly, the focus is not on Alex in labor. The labor here is Larry's and that of his male assistant, who perform the surgery to extract the child, and the product of this technological labor of men is appropriated by them as the money they gain by selling their research to a pharmaceutical company that is going to produce the drug to be used by, or on, women. What seems like a good deed—Alex is endangering his life to help women prevent miscarriages—also creates conditions for more of women's reproductive labor being controlled by men. And while Diana does get the child, the only way she can profit from the research project that relied on her egg appropriation is via being a wife of Alex.

The claim to child ownership by the head of the lab introduces yet another layer of assisted reproduction consequences. The head of the lab appears on the scene just as Alex tells Diana that he is pregnant because he is testing the drug on himself. When Alex tells her it is her egg, she becomes livid. "*My* Junior?" she asks. "*Our* Junior now," Alex responds. Diana reacts to this appropriation with a diatribe that outlines its risks for women; she calls it "an utterly immoral, selfish, arrogant stunt without any regard for [her] feelings whatsoever" that is "just so male." She says, "What did you think you were doing? You think men don't hold enough cards? You have to take this away from us as well? . . . It's pitiful." What may seem like an overreaction is confirmed, however, as a warranted response to a legitimate threat. The conversation between Alex and Diana is interrupted by the head of the lab, who arrives to claim both the baby and pregnant Alex as the property of the lab. Because the experiment was conducted with the use of the university's resources, it owns the results. The personhood of ART-conceived people and people who physically labor (Alex in the film, but women in the real world) to bring them into being becomes uncertain in the context where technological means and aspects of reproduction permeate but are thought of as separate from the natural act of conception and birth. Within such framework, the relationship between biology and science implies that biology is the experimental subject that can be manipulated and owned by those who control technology and fund scientific research. *Junior* does not dwell in this rather scary possibility too long and erases it through defeating the comedic villain. When the security guards want to escort Alex to the ambulance, and Diana, who steps in to protect him, is easily pushed away, Alex shoves the head of the lab much more forcefully to protect her and the baby. As a "good patriarchal man," he defends his family and his child from the violence of other men but also from the encroachment of technoscientific discourse that aims to recast him and the baby as research subjects. The film reestablishes their human status by showing Alex as the patriarchal protector of a family that begins to look more and more like a regular heterocoital one, regardless of who is carrying the child.

A struggle that is less noticeably ominous (because it is often funny) occurs consistently in the film over the appropriation of feminist discourse. When Alex is fighting the head of the lab and the security guards, he declares, "My body. My choice!" He is claiming his reproductive rights, but the slogan that has been historically used to advocate for women's reproductive freedom and bodily autonomy sounds questionable following Diana's outline of the consequences of female alienation from child gestation and labor. When Alex shares with Larry that Diana said that they "had taken away her dignity and the sacred role of womanhood," Larry dismisses this concern by saying that pregnant women always complain that they wish men tried carrying children. "You finally do it and what do you get? Attitude and insults," he says reducing a grave concern to a gender stereotype. After Alex escapes from the head of the lab and goes into hiding in the home for expectant mothers, reappropriation of feminist thinking accompanies his transformation and works to universalize and relativize reproductive labor's significance. At a group discussion of fears expectant mothers share, the leader says, "We have to dispense with the myth that some are born with the maternal instinct and others are not." Since this statement is not explicitly about women, Alex's presence among the audience opens a space for imagining male pregnancy as a fact of life. The words may simultaneously imply that he is one of those with the maternal instinct and that no one is really born with one. Either way, he is not that different from women, and what he is doing can be considered natural. The group leader follows with a pronatalist remark that invokes a blurred gender boundary and paves an even firmer way toward Alex's inclusion: "The little girl tending her doll collection is no more a natural-born mother than the tomboy down the street." Finally, she proclaims, "There is no standard. There are no naturals." At this moment, Diana arrives, just in time to catch the tenor of the conversation and begin to worry about the consequences of her alienation from the reproductive process. The statements that are meant to comfort and inspire confidence in women who are doubting their compliance to the cultural standards of motherhood now become more overt harbingers of their potential disempowerment.

Alienation of women from the reproductive process in the context of ARTs also emerges in *Delivery Man,* which leans on the absence or superficial treatment of women characters as a way of dealing with the consequences of sperm donation. The anxiety over uncertain paternity heightened by the process of sperm-donor conception is handled in the film by doubling down on connecting the biological fatherhood to the social one and focusing on the significance of knowing one's biological father. Keeping the focus on the biological father is helped by the removal of the mothers and extended families of donor-conceived children from the picture. Unlike the horror genre, which resorts to the monstrous feminine trope, comedy is figuring out the way to live with sperm-alienation anxieties. *Delivery Man* does it through erasure of women who use the alienated sperm for their purposes. The focus on the main character and sperm donor David, and specifically on normalizing his fatherhood of hundreds of children within the heterocoital framework, shows the elasticity of the patriarchal discourse that aims to retain power over the reproductive landscape by insisting on traditional ideas of parenthood even in the contexts where they appear ridiculous and impossible.

The normalization of David's situation is facilitated by a traditional rom com plot that shows a transformation of a developmentally arrested male into a responsible adult who finally accepts heteronormative responsibilities. The film opens with credits over a sequence of frames capturing the decor of David's apartment, which looks rather like a teenager's room and suggests a lack of adult responsibilities. We see toys, traffic signs, a foosball table, overdue bills, photos with many different women, dried cannabis plants, and so on. The theme of immaturity is reinforced by David's continuous presentation as a failure. He is in debt after investing eighty thousand dollars in a Ponzi scheme. He borrowed the money from thugs who are now after him. He is trying to make money to pay them back by growing hydroponic pot, but he cannot take care of plants. His pregnant girlfriend, Emma, tells him that she will have the child on her own because he "disappears," is "unreliable," "ha[s] money problems," and, overall, doesn't "have a life." His life, in other words, is not a life a man of his age should lead. The arc of the film is David's transformation from a good-natured but pathetic loser into a father figure responsible not only for his biological child heterocoitally conceived with Emma, but for the children conceived with his sperm donations. His transformation is facilitated by his anonymous reconnecting with some of the children who want to know him and then coming out as Starbuck (his donor nickname).

David's character develops against two foils—his brother, Aleksy (Bobby Moynihan), who is about to have a child with his wife (never shown), and his friend and lawyer, Brett (Chris Pratt), a father of four children, who seems to be their primary caregiver and whose wife is never shown either. Both Aleksy and Brett advise David not to have children. In the first scenes of the film, Aleksy, who is driven crazy by his pregnant wife's moods and desires, tells David, "Do not procreate, David. Reproduction is a very bad idea. Do not reproduce ever." When David is sharing with Brett that he was "in shock" at first when Emma told him she was pregnant, but after the fear went away, he felt that "this could be the most beautiful thing that ever happened" to him, Brett urges him to convince Emma to get an abortion. The reasons for this stance become clear as all his four children, who are supposed to be in bed, appear during his and David's conversation in the backyard and challenge his authority by disobeying his "go to bed" and "don't do this" instructions. Three boys lie down to sleep in the sandbox, and the daughter slaps his face, repeating, "Daddy! Daddy!" but not saying what she wants. He is clearly emasculated by his children, who do not listen to him. Brett is trying to disabuse David of his desire to have a child by explaining that fatherhood is disempowering, his freedom will be over, and that the children are "a black hole" that will "suck up all [his] energy." On top of that, David "[doesn't] have the skills to bring up a child." David, however, still imagines that a child can bring "order" to his life or, in other words, give his life meaning.

As the plot develops, Aleksy and Brett serve to bring attention to specific aspects of David's fatherhood. Aleksy's pride in his newborn son's pooping is mirrored by the fatherly pride David feels when he discovers that one of his donor-conceived children is a major-league basketball player. In contrast to Aleksy, however, David's character is developed further through his anonymous encounters with donor-conceived children who are less successful. He helps a struggling actor child to get a role by lending him his truck to go to an audition, contributes to a drug-addicted daughter's recovery, and spends time with a severely disabled child who has been placed in assisted living and seems abandoned by his family. Through these encounters, David is becoming a more complex character and a more caring, responsible man. His care is, however, different from the consistent daily childcare Brett provides to his children. Brett's implied emasculation by the need to tend to children in the absence of his wife contrasts David's heroic swooping in and saving his children. After he has acquainted himself with about ten of them, he tells Brett that he "had an epiphany" that he cannot be the father of 533 children, but he can be "their guardian angel." This happens while Brett is packing school lunches, an act of care that seems pedestrian next to David's heroics. As the voice of reason, Brett points to David's narcissism and suggests an insanity plea in the lawsuit that 142 of the donor-conceived children have launched to deanonymize David. The film, however, doubles down on the heroics and shows David saving even his heterocoital child. After the first ultrasound, David talks Emma out of a potential abortion. While Emma is watching children at the playground, she is having second thoughts. Slowly and forcefully, David says to her, "You are going to be a good mother." She is immediately convinced and lets him be a "father on probation," which he joyfully accepts.

Throughout the film, David is positioned, albeit not very convincingly to a critical viewer, as an increasingly complex, caring man who can take control not only of his own life but also the lives of his children. *He* is shown as the connective tissue between the children, not their mothers, and not even the children themselves. As he is following yet another of his biological sons, he accidentally walks into a meeting of all the children participating in the lawsuit to deanonymize Starbuck. When he realizes where he is, he slowly turns his head to the side, and the camera shows five young men sitting to his left. He turns back, and the camera lingers on his face, now aligned with the young men's like a stroboscopic image or a vanishing point, suggestive of continuity and similarity (see figure 3.3). He turns to the right, stands up, looks around, and sees more young men and women. Because everyone

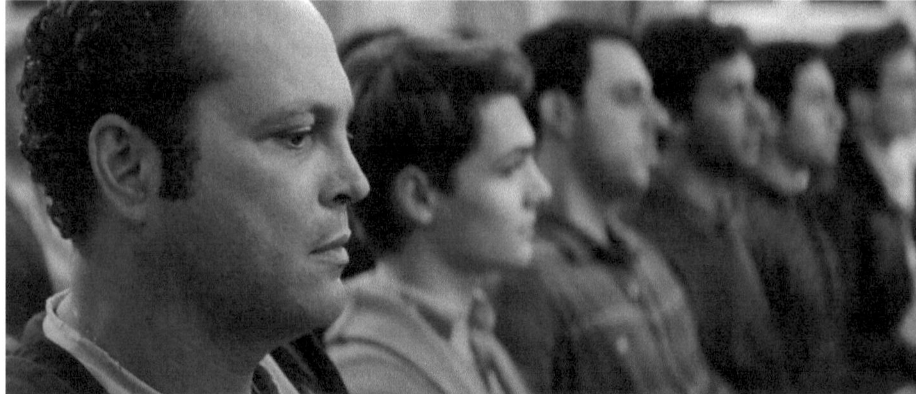

FIGURE 3.3. David and his donor-conceived children in *Delivery Man*. Walt Disney Studios Motion Pictures, 2013.

thinks he has stood up to speak, he has to deliver a speech in which he suggests that their acquaintance with each other is already family-making, even if they do not know who the father is. But this scene looks formal in contrast to the conversation he later has in the hallway with all the children that he is now acquainted with personally. He says that he is the adoptive father of Ryan, the disabled child, and is attending the event on his behalf. As he gets recognized by more of the children, he introduces them to each other, creating a more intimate circle and reinforcing the idea that he is the link in the chain that connects them all to each other. In this and several other scenes, the film reimagines the man as the source of both biological and sociocultural continuity, thus introducing a revision of male reproductive consciousness by stitching gendered distinctions as theorized by O'Brien. This continuity and connectedness is maintained by the film's focus on David's interactions with a limited group of children and implicit extrapolation of the possibility of such relationship to all 533. The impossibility of being a "good father" to this number of children is masked by David's personal confidence and by substituting grand gestures, as expressions of social fatherhood, for the everyday process of childcare.

David's paternalistic narcissism is fed by his father, the voice of the old patriarchy. While Aleksy and Brett, who participate in daily childcare, can be seen as representatives of the more modern kind of fatherhood, David's father is portrayed as a provider responsible for the well-being of their family and business. He misses his late wife, who seems to have been the source of the family's emotional cohesion. Now this function is performed by her portrait on the wall, overlooking the daily life of her family. When David outs himself to his father as the sperm donor and asks for advice on how a "normal person" would behave in this situation, his father says that such a person would not be in David's situation. To David's "What would my brothers do?" he responds, "Your brothers are not mentally equipped to deal with a situation like this" and makes him feel special for being "one of the few people on this Earth able to deal with [this]." David's father implies that David can do it due to his generosity and care for others—for example, he used the money earned for sperm donations to send his parents on their dream vacation. Such big-heartedness, which allegedly makes David equipped to be a father to many children, has led him, however, to reckless financial decisions that undermine his ability to provide for his family with Emma. In response to David's flunking this requirement of the patriarchy, David's conversation with his father redefines the role of the patriarchal man as the family provider. The father expresses regret for not spending more time with his family and offers David his share of inheritance so he could pay off his debt. This takes care of the moral dilemma David has been struggling with. He has won some money in a countersuit to protect his anonymity, and he could use this money to pay off his debt. But now he wants to reveal his identity to the biological children, and this means he loses the money. With his father's inheritance, he does not have to make a choice between being a known father of 533 children or starting his heterocoital family with Emma on a strong financial footing. The traditional father-provider thus endorses David's sentimental fatherhood by confirming that it is important to be there emotionally for children. When David doubts his competency at fatherhood, his father helps him see the difference between being an incompetent worker (which David is) and being a man whom "everyone loves." A social father is an object of love that just needs to be known in order to fulfill his role.

This idea is echoed in the testimonies of the children, who explain the need to know the identity of their donor. The children's lawsuit claim is based on the "basic human right to know who their biological father is,"[15] and their testimonies speak of the father as a formative presence that can shape the course of their life just by being known. Without such a figure, the film implies, the "children [are] lost in the wilderness." The musician child, for instance, says, "when I write music, I write it because . . ."—he trails off, but the audience is invited to connect the dots and assume that his inspiration comes from knowing that his father is out there. A lot of the children speak of the father as a vital ingredient to their sense of selfhood: "You know, it's central to who

15. This right is not stated in these terms in the United Nations' declaration of human rights, but the right to know parents "as far as possible" is stated in the resolution 44/25 of the 1989 Convention on the Rights of the Child, https://www.ohchr.org/en/instruments-mechanisms/instruments/convention-rights-child.

I am. It's really all I've thought about"; "I just want to feel like I have a part of myself"; "I would like to meet the guy, the man who created me." Some children do imagine the father as doing care work that could have made their life better. Young Boozer, who is an alcoholic, attributes his issues to his father's absence: "I know how, for me, I wasn't actually able to grow up with a dad." The drug-addicted daughter implies the need of paternal support at challenging junctures of her life, as she says, "And there's a lot of transitions in my life that I've come across." In her case, as in some others', David's appearance in her life actually "resolved" her issues with drug addiction; she is now clean. David's "magical power" to fix his children's problems by performing discreet acts of care as a guardian angel seems to suggest a questionable equivalency between the labor of consistent care needed to raise a child and fatherhood as just "being there" or "being known."

The equivalency between David's heterocoital and donor fatherhoods is suggested in other ways as well. David misses his heterocoital child's birth, which equalizes his experiences—he has not been there for the births of any of his children. In this case, we are invited to extrapolate into the donorship context the heterocoital understanding that not being there for the birth of a child does not make someone less of a father if their biological paternity checks out. When David goes to see Emma in the hospital after she gives birth, he is told by the nurse, "Your family is here to see you." It turns out that it is his biological brothers and father plus the donor-conceived children. After he addresses this new family configuration and apologizes for lying to them, they all hug him. He acknowledges that "this is weird," referring to the number of family members and the mix of his heterocoital and donor-conceived biological lineages. But what seems even more weird is the shortage of women in this picture; the camera frames generations of fathers and their children as "the family," suggesting that women might be tangential to the portrayed continuity. David negotiates his moral right to such continuity in his conversation with Emma at the hospital. He leads with "Will you marry me?" When she agrees, he confesses he is Starbuck. Her reaction is to deny him fatherhood: "This is no longer your child." We know why she thinks it is not normal, based on an earlier scene in a baby supply store when they discussed Starbuck without her knowing who he is. David was trying to defend him, but she parried by asking the salesperson if they had a stroller for 533 children. With this question, she emphasized that it is humanly impossible to provide necessary care to 533 children. David shuts her objections down by delivering "two points."

The first one is that he is changing and that "it's not anyone but [him] who can decide if [he is] the father or not. Not a judge, not my family, not

Dr. Phil, and in the end, not you." In other words, nobody but the father can decide if he is the father or not. Here David delivers an interesting negotiation of known paternity. He is rejecting social ways of establishing paternity (he does not mention DNA tests), and the proclamation he makes establishes the man's decision as the sole basis of paternity and fatherhood. He does not appeal to biology, genetics, or the heterocoital act, and by omitting these, he is establishing a rule of patriarchy that allows him to claim his progeny because he said so. It is understood that he is claiming the children genetically related to him, and this implication grounds his ambition within the patriarchal discourse, making the transition to the next level less transgressive. But casting this claim as a social one normalizes appropriation of the multiple non-heterocoital but biogenetic progeny through means other than the nuclear family. Such appropriation implies a redistribution of reproductive labor to the families who used sperm donations. When he tries to sell the idea to Emma, he mentions "vast amounts of free babysitting," that is, he is imagining fatherhood not as a challenge to his resources but a gain from his children, who are now supposed to fulfill a family obligation. As a typical patriarchal man to whom family is a source of free unacknowledged labor, he appears oblivious to the cost to others of his ambition. He believes that there are "a few drawbacks" and a "tremendous amount of joy" in this situation and thinks that his "risking all" for the sake of 533 children should convince Emma that he is going to be there for her and their heterocoital child. No acknowledgment is given to the majority of the donor-conceived children, who did not want to know his identity, nor to the fact that he may be less present in the lives of his heterocoital family if his donor-conceived children need his help. The whole project seems to be based on David's megalomania, which makes him think that what he is doing is important, "like the first steps on the Moon," because "no one on this planet has ever experienced it before." The second point he is making in his argument attempting to convince Emma to allow him to be her husband and the father of their child is that his marriage proposal is not "a scam" and he needs her in his life. Unbelievably, such statement seems to be enough. She kisses him, and all issues seem to be resolved. After that, she shows their son, through the glass door of the hospital room, to all the donor-conceived children—the baby's introduction to the family signals her acceptance of the situation.

The last scene of the film is a montage of David's split-second interactions with some of the donor conceived children, showing him as a useful father whose (often ridiculous) advice is appreciated by his children. "Many thanks from your entire *real* family," says the last child he hugs. In lived relationships between donors, recipients, donor-conceived children, and involved extended families, negotiations of belonging and kinship are typically more complex, varied, and multi-nodal, even within the heterocoital family framework (Nordqvist and Gilman, 2022). *Delivery Man* forgoes such complexities. It makes knowledge of genetic paternity sufficient for making a family "real." And while it still relies on the nuclear family metaphor to restore the donor-father to full fatherhood (still understood as biological and social), the social aspect of fatherhood is crystallized into the concept of biogenetic paternity knowledge that makes a child "whole" and creates a sense of biocultural continuity. It may not seem so different from how the heterocoital framework works, until we consider that the technological means that help establish genetic paternity, and lay claim to child ownership, make institutions such as marriage and monogamy, as well as heterocoitus as a point of origin, tangential or unnecessary for establishing known paternity and for mediation of men's relationship with species continuity and futurity. In other words, the ways of controlling women's reproductive power are in flux. This is not to say that heterocoital cultures are going to disappear any time soon from our lives or imaginations, but it does open possibilities for revisions of the patriarchy that may not revise its main tenet: the power of men over women and children. The following chapter looks at sci-fi texts that explore some of such possibilities.

CHAPTER 4

Adoption and ARTs in Science Fiction

Reproductive Futurities

> The sense of delegitimation can make it harder to sustain a bond, a bond that is not real anyway, a bond that does not "exist," that never had a chance to exist, that was never meant to exist. If you're not real, it can be hard to sustain yourselves over time.
>
> —Judith Butler, *Undoing Gender* (114)

The 2021 TV show *Foundation,* based on a science fiction book series by Isaac Asimov, features a clone dynasty ruling the twelve-thousand-year-old Galactic Empire. At any given time, three clones of Cleon I, the founder of the Empire, are alive: Brother Dawn, Brother Day, and Brother Dusk (see figure 4.1). They do not have individual names and are distinguished by their age range. Brother Day rules as emperor, while brother Dawn is learning, and retired brother Dusk is assisting. The clones are meant to represent a single person living the stages of his life over and over. To assure consistency of the image, they work on looking and moving alike. At a dinner scene, they are shown performing even such small movements as lifting a glass in perfect synchronicity. While they have unique personality traits and interests, all three present to the public as the same person. The unity of identity demonstrates genealogical continuity of power consolidated in a single person, Cleon I, whose legacy the clones preserve as they expand and control the Empire. There is no mention of who brings them to life, and no mother figure except for an AI that looks like a woman and acts like an assistant rather than a caregiver. The clones are reproductively self-sufficient and thus represent a triumph of autonomous male reproduction, which goes hand in hand with an unprecedented consolidation of patriarchal power that assures the stability of the Empire. The introduction of clones in the TV show narrative is a departure from Asimov's book series. Cloning is not part of the original storylines,

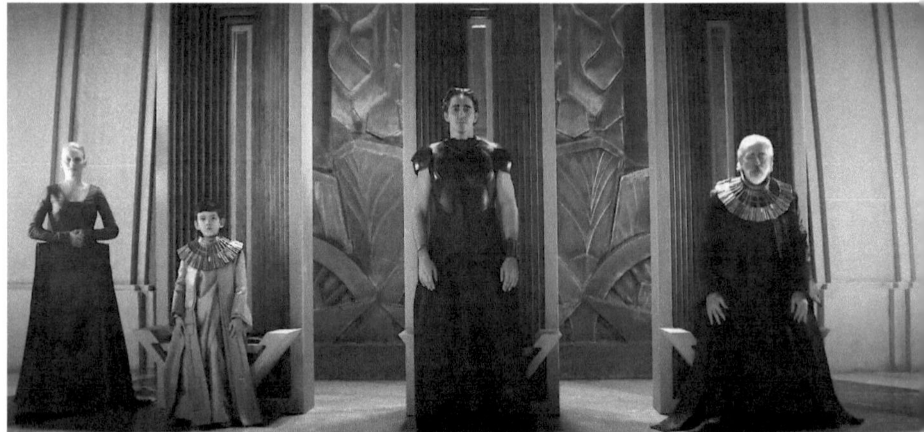

FIGURE 4.1. The genetic dynasty of clones in *Foundation*. Skydance Television, 2021.

and it seems possible that the clones' appearance reflects more contemporary cultural concerns with reproductive technologies finding their way into the show's creators' imaginations. It is also peculiar that the representation of clones is not used to suggest stagnation and an evolutionary dead end as is common in clone narratives.[1] The clones' permanence and sameness are ideologically repurposed as political stability achieved through the reproduction of authoritarianism that assures the Empire's progress in space colonization and technological development.

The representation of clones in *Foundation* abandons cultural dressing-up of assisted reproduction as heterocoital and offers a radical conceptualization of male reproductive consciousness in a context where it no longer has to contend with the need for a woman's body as a reproductive resource.[2] It is a departure from representations that reveal the attempts of patriarchy to reinstate the man in the reproductive process and species continuity through reimagining technoreproduction as heterocoital. So far, we have observed how heterocoital imaginary may subsume challenges to it by "inventing" coitus as long as the man's genetic material becomes part of the child. Discourses of adoption, and some forms of ARTs that lend themselves to such cultural mediation, reinscribe the logic of heterocoitus on reproductive technologies due to the patriarchal inertia that demands that the new form of reproduction "match" the institutions and social structures the child is born into.

1. Season 2 introduces such scenes, but their analysis is beyond the scope of this book.

2. Season 2 of *Foundation* engages with this concern, along the lines of analysis in this book. Since the manuscript production process started before season 2 was released, its analysis is beyond the scope of this book.

Foundation, however, toys with a form of ART that transcends the heterocoital coupling (like, for example, in vitro gametogenesis) and has the potential to disrupt the structures of both male and female reproductive consciousnesses. It offers a glimpse of an alternative way for the patriarchy to survive in the world of non-heterocoital reproduction—by purging the woman from reproduction and redefining reproductive capability, coupled with alienation from reproductive process and species continuity as a privileged state. In the show's imagination, brother Day's biological immortality and full patriarchal control over reproduction amplify the focus on mortality as an instrument of political power. Brother Day (Lee Pace) destroys the population of a whole planet with a flick of his fingers to eliminate a perceived threat to the Empire. He sacrifices millions for the sake of political continuity that assures immortality to his dynasty. This mass execution demonstrates the consequences of the unrevised and universalized reproductive consciousness described by O'Brien as male, alienated, and tethered to Heideggerian *Dasein*—a conceptualization of "human temporality" characterized by male fixation on death as "the proper vantage point" (Brodribb 257). *Foundation* toys with an extreme appropriation of assisted reproduction by patriarchy, which may seem implausibly apocalyptic. However, it very plausibly suggests that the future of heteropatriarchy may become open to revisions due to the consequences of assisted reproduction, and that such revisions may not necessarily move us toward more freedom. The films and TV shows discussed in this chapter engage with the instabilities and imagined possibilities for revisions of reproduction. They show the significance of our ideas about universal features of human reproduction as a measure of humanity and personhood and alert us to the need for interventions in the construction of the future reproductive landscape.

To explore the ways Western cultures imagine reproductive futurities, it would make sense to turn to science fiction—a genre and a mode that Sherryl Vint describes as a "toolbox of methods for conceptualizing, intervening in, and living through rapid and widespread sociotechnical change" (158).[3] Science fiction seems to be a fitting medium for examining cultural narratives that try on different forms of "signification" (Squier 16) for new kinds of identities and relatedness in a time when the reproductive process is undergoing change. Kinship that ceases being stitched together by biogenetic relatedness grounded in heterocoitus loses its moorings because biology is exposed as an unreliable anchor of human identity. It does not become less biological and

3. See also Jelača; Braidotti (2006) for validations of sci-fi as methodology for exploring "changes and transformations . . . in our posthuman present" (Braidotti, qtd. in Jelača 383).

somehow more cultural. Instead, biology itself becomes or begins to be more universally understood as "a complex cultural practice" (Haraway 1996, 336). That is why there emerges a need for new narratives: to make sense of new kinds of biological relatedness. In *Liminal Lives,* Susan Merrill Squier draws on Latour's understanding of scientific discourse as narrative and considers fiction "as a technology of signification, generating biocultural meanings from the new technologies of recombination" (Squier 16). Fiction becomes the grounds on which the tug-of-war between emergent meanings of reproductive technologies and the imposition of heterocoital imaginary on new reproductive possibilities is carried out. We can already see that some ARTs have become subjects of realistic film genres, like drama, which signals their growing acceptance and shows that their strangeness can be subsumed within the heterocoital reproduction metaphors. Other, less easily co-opted ways of reproduction may remain subjects of speculative genres, where alternatives to traditional ways of understanding reproduction, origin, kinship, and belonging are still being negotiated. In such narratives, the established biocultural connections may be destabilized enough for heteropatriarchy to undergo some liberating revisions, but the desired revisions are only possibilities, not guarantees. But speculative genres help us understand what is at stake when technological interventions in human reproduction destabilize the boundary between humans and nonhumans and disturb the consensus around the definition of humanity that insists on seeing technology as the Other.

A.I. Artificial Intelligence, an adoption narrative of a robot boy placed in a human family, which this book opened with, is a cinematic sci-fi text rich in evidence of the way our human imaginary may construct the meaning of difference between humans and nonhumans based on their origin. It is an example of how a humanlike being, for whom technology is a vital part of their emergence and becoming, may be denied acceptance, as suspect, into cultures built on the heterocoital order. David (Haley Joel Osment) is built as an eight-year-old with the body and range of expression virtually indistinguishable from an organic human. He is created by the roboticist Hobby (William Hurt) in the likeness of his dead son, David, and is adopted by Monica and Henry Swinton (Frances O'Connor and Sam Robards) as a substitute for their incurably ill biological son, Martin (Jake Thomas), who has been cryogenically frozen. Adoptive father Henry believes that a robot child, programmed to experience love for a human in the same way a child loves a parent, can serve as a transitional object and help Monica to deal with the pending loss of Martin. As an engineer, he only sees in David a high-functioning robot, and he never develops a close relationship with him. For Hobby, who wrote the book *What Will Make a Robot Human?,* David is an experiment in creating a robot that aspires to the human condition. Hobby is testing a robot's capacity to love beyond its programmed set of outward manifestations and verbal expressions. By programming David to love a parent as a child would and placing him with the Swintons, Hobby hopes to create conditions under which David can develop "a kind of subconscious"—"an inner world of metaphor, of intuition," that will give the robot the humanlike ability to "chase down [his] dreams," "inspired by love" and "fueled by desire." In other words, Hobby believes that a placement with a heterosexual nuclear family can help develop a robot's consciousness enough to share and become part of the human imaginary, which is something that no robot has ever achieved before. Hobby believes that the ability to dream is co-emergent with experiencing love as a mystery—the way it is felt by humans. He also seems to believe that family is the source of such experiences and that the purest form of love is the unconditional love of a child for a parent. However, Hobby's enthusiasm for his new project is checked by a question from one of his colleagues. She asks, "Can we get a human to love him back?" and introduces the main conflict of the film: can a loving robot achieve the condition of full "human intelligibility" (Butler 118) and become a legitimate subject who can be taken up into the structures of human feelings as an equal? The film explores this conflict through David's relationship with his adoptive human mother.

Monica herself is not part of the adoption decision process. She is presented with David and given a choice of activating his "irreversible" imprinting on her as a "mommy," if and when she feels ready for it. Unlike Hobby and Henry, for whom David is an experiment, Monica seems to be drawn into a more intimate relationship with David. Her confusion over what he is—"He is—He's so real—But he's not. . . . But outside he just looks so real. Like he is a child—a child"—makes him uncanny to her at first and an object of maternal desire later. Eventually, she activates his imprinting, and he becomes even more childlike and humanlike. He is eager to please her to secure her love, and the expression of his emotions becomes more fluid. Haley Joel Osment's acting loses the jerky moves and unnatural turns of the head that reveal his character's robotic build, and David's difference from an organic eight-year-old boy becomes a memory in the mind of a viewer rather than a quality invoked by repeated visual signification. Such erasure of visible difference adds more poignancy to the moments in which his mecha build becomes apparent again, but it also tests the viewer's and the film's human characters' ability to forget and to see David as a human child as the film works through the meaning of this difference.

When Martin is brought back after a cure for his disease becomes available, David's difference becomes a contested condition around which his belonging with the adoptive human family is negotiated. The problem is presented to David when Monica introduces Martin to him as "my son," not "your brother," and when Martin explains to him that he is a "new super toy," like the walking and talking toy bear Teddy, but not "real" like Martin. David's role in the family is also redefined after Martin's return: he is there to keep Martin company and help Monica care for her recovering orga son. A change in his status suggests that he has been treated as a substitute who has become unnecessary after the original was reinstated in his family role. But David, who developed the need to be loved in return by his human mother (fulfilling both Hobby's and his doubting colleague's expectations), is frustrated by this change. His desire for his mother's love grows in proportion to Monica's withdrawal, and his way of securing her love becomes the dogged striving to become "real." In this way, the film evokes the cruel question that still haunts adoption, "Can you love like your own a nonbiologically related child?" while it prompts us to examine what counts as real kinship and who is entitled to being taken up into its structures as a real subject. The answer the film provides is elusive. David's desire to become real turns into a quest in which his only hope is the transformative magic of the Blue Fairy—a character from *Pinocchio,* which Monica reads to the boys before bed. Martin chooses the book to cruelly remind David that he is a toy, but what matters to David is the possibility to become "real" by meeting the Blue Fairy and becoming a "real boy." It is not quite clear, though, what "real" means in this context, and while the film offers a few explanations, it never settles on a firmly defined condition that would make David real. Instead, it offers several possibilities that are simultaneously at work.

Most obviously, David's concerns about being "real" may have to do with different qualities of his mechanical versus human organic embodiment—a difference that underscores the absence of shared vulnerabilities and common origins. Several scenes suggest that David's belonging in the Swintons' family hinges on the kind of body he has and the way the humans perceive it. For example, Monica is pulled into a mother-son relationship with him because he looks real enough for her to imagine him as her son. She decides to activate the imprinting protocol after she witnesses his ability to laugh at the things humans find funny. But she is unsettled when David picks up the phone and turns his body into a receiver as he transmits the voices of Henry and his assistant: he looks possessed. Such sudden exposures of David's body's different functionality breach the illusion and remind us of his nonhumanity. The robotic difference is underscored when Martin bases his claim to being real on his *in*ability to do "power stuff" like walking on the ceiling or flying—things that, he imagines, David can do. And even though David cannot do such things, the durability of his body—"never ill"—stands out in contrast when Martin arrives home from the hospital wearing an oxygen mask and slumped in a wheelchair, obviously vulnerable. Throughout the film, David's body is presented as at once more durable than a human's, and more vulnerable. Yet its vulnerability is always suspect because it is not vulnerable in a human way. The result is that David's outward resemblance to humans does not always evoke feelings of affinity or empathy; when the difference of his body from a human's is exposed, it becomes, in Masahiro Mori's sense, uncanny. Masahiro, a Japanese robotics scientist, developed the theory of the "uncanny valley"—a dip in the graph that represents the degree of a human's feeling of affinity with a robot relative to the degree of the robot's human likeness. The graph shows that while our affinity with robots grows as their design becomes more and more humanlike, when the robot begins to approach 100 percent resemblance to a human but does not yet look human enough, we find it uncanny and may react with fear and disgust. We may experience a similar revulsion when an entity we believed to be human reveals its nonhuman qualities, like in David's case.

David's nonhuman vulnerability is exposed when the rivalry between David and Martin prompts David to respond to Martin's taunts and eat spinach during family dinner. David sees eating as a way to claim belonging like Martin's: "real boys" can eat. But David breaks because steamed spinach destroys his circuits. To feel sympathy and be able to hold his hand during the repair "surgery," Monica has to overcome the horror she feels observing the summoned repairmen struggling to clear out green goop from David's exposed innards while he is fully awake and smiling at her reassuringly. His attempt to belong by doing what "a real boy" does alienates him instead: humans understand that although capable of breaking down, he can be repaired, and that he is not alive, and therefore vulnerable to the inevitability of death, in the same way humans are. David's humanlike embodiment is thus exposed as not real but instead a way to make him appear more humanlike and seduce humans into feeling and caring for him like they would for a human child.

Such illusion makes him dangerous because he may not be able to empathetically understand the limits of the human body even though he can be programmed to recognize and react to pain stimuli. At Martin's birthday party, when a boy points a knife at David's arm trying to find out if he can feel pain, David reacts in a programmed way: he seeks safety like a human child would. He hides behind Martin, hugs him, and starts backing away from the boy with the knife, pleading, "Keep me safe! Keep me safe!" David and Martin accidentally fall into the swimming pool and go under water, but David does not unclasp his grip. He has to be pried away from Martin. In this instance,

David's programmed performance of humanlike vulnerability actually endangers the life of Martin, whose vulnerability is a natural, inescapable condition. The difference of David's vulnerability excludes him from human consideration when the life of a human is at stake: Martin is saved and David is left at the bottom of the pool. In the eyes of humans, he is not one of them, not alive and thus not worthy of saving.

These scenes locate David's (robotic) difference in embodiment and suggest that "real boys" who deserve the love and care of their families need a certain kind of body. Joshua Knobe, an experimental philosopher with an interest in cognitive science, shows that human willingness to assume that an entity is capable of experiencing cognitive and phenomenal states similar to ours—to think and feel, or in other words, to be like us—depends not only on this entity's observed behavior but on "whether the entity has the right sort of *body*" (187). While we have no problem imagining a disembodied entity, such as a corporation, or a robotic entity made of silicon and metal, capable of "deciding, intending, knowing," Knobe says, "something about the presence of our faces, our flesh, our biological nature, must be triggering people to think that we have phenomenal consciousness"—a precondition for the ability to feel and experience phenomenal states like pain or pleasure (190–91). These observations may suggest humans believe that only the "right sort" of body can empathize with human emotions and phenomenal states. But entities with which we do not recognize shared, animal nature may not share our affective and phenomenal experience and vulnerabilities. Therefore, they are not like us and may be dangerous to us because they may not be capable of empathy and a relationship of reciprocal care guided by the "golden rule." The swimming pool scene shows that even though David is programmed to behave like a human, and his body is outwardly indistinguishable from a human's, it is not always possible to predict what he might do because his mecha embodiment may lead to a behavior that humans cannot anticipate based on their own experience. The invisibility of his difference makes this danger even more menacing. But it also suggests that to be recognized as human, it is not enough for the body to look like a human one. Children at the pool party, who have not seen proof of David's mecha build but only *know* that he is mecha, do not think of him as one of them, even though the appearance of his body is indistinguishable from theirs. The right kind of body, in this context, means not just the one that appears human but the one of common ancestry—genetically human, sharing a universal kind of origin, and belonging to the same species—the one that guarantees shared ontology through known genealogy.

Cultural preoccupation with known genealogy, well established in the context of adoption, shows that the belief in originary continuity as a condition for being taken up into the human structures of feeling and considered "one of our own" may be present even in nonbiological kinship as "the fantasy of the genetic that continues to haunt [the adoption's] desire to deessentialize the family and to make it into the 'mere' experience of relationality" (Jerng 2010, 234). In *Claiming Others,* Mark Jerng shows that "the desire for biological relations is constructed" by adoptive and biological families through "the drive to produce [physical] 'likeness'" as a measure of unity (211). Such unity depends on "the certainty of the biological constitution of family, an essential, noncontingent connection to other people" (216). In adoption, physical likeness or family narratives of intergenerational quirks and behaviors that are imagined as biologically inherited may operate as a sign of known origin, continuous with ancestors and descendants, which provides an assurance that the family has reproduced a child of their own kind. In David's case, manipulating his embodiment successfully to perform genealogical continuity with the Swintons (as an adoptee would be compelled to do) becomes impossible. He cannot clear the hurdle of his known nonhuman, non-heterocoital, manufactured origin and therefore cannot be imagined functioning as one's own human child.

David's becoming real is impossible in a culture that imagines its reproduction as heterocoital reproduction of heterosexual bodies that get socialized through the oedipal script. Anyone who is perceived as unable to complete oedipalization (as, for example, in the case of asexual reproduction when the biological origin is unknown, different, or nonexistent and the ability to trace the "kind" that is reproduced is diluted) would have trouble securing a place within the heterocoital symbolic order as a fully recognized person. By functioning as a child, David helps Monica and Harry maintain a resemblance to a human family. He makes Monica look like a mother again. But he is not their own child who can reproduce "their own kind," because he does not have the right kind of body, which can grow up, achieve heterosexuality through oedipalization, and reproduce humans heterocoitally. As such, Monica and the rest of the family cannot imagine him in the social position of the "real son." In turn, the presence of such an entity within a human family would be "a form of derealization" for this family (Butler 114).

The doubt that David can become "real" by entering the heterocoital symbolic order is expressed in the questions asked by Hobby's colleague: "Can you get a human to love the robot back?" or, rephrased, "If a robot could genuinely love a person, what responsibility does that person hold toward that mecha in return?" These questions aim to reveal a presumption that a robot is not a person and that it does not deserve to be included into the systems of human relations as a subject with rights. They may also imply that human personhood is the precondition for being genuinely loved and cared for. The woman who asks this question is interested in whether a robot can be a person. But Hobby does not seem to understand the meaning of the question he is asked. His experiment pursues a different question, articulated in the title of his book *What Will Make a Robot Human?*, and he seems to be oblivious to the contradictions that robotic, manufactured origin may present to someone who is trying to achieve humanity "the human way." Hobby believes that David can become human if he develops a subconscious and will be able to desire not what he is told but what he wants, and to "chase dreams" to make them reality, like humans do. But this vision of the robot as a liberal-humanist autonomous subject is undermined by Hobby speaking of David as a machine with specific functionality that "will not only open up a completely new market; it will fill a great human need" felt by many childless couples who do not qualify for a child license in the resource-depleted world of the future. His "little mecha" is conceived to be "caught in a freeze-frame," "never changing," following an exclusive imprinting protocol that would not let the robot transfer its love onto another love object. David's capacity for free will ends up locked within the desire to become real by becoming a real son, but the route which could take him there is closed off to him because of his origin and cultural ideas about how heterocoital origin and oedipalization produce human persons.

In other words, David is an entity that, in the words of Rosi Braidotti, is "not . . . fully human"—what women and enslaved people used to be and children still are—the kind that would be aspiring to and experiencing the human condition with no claim to full human freedom and rights (2013, 1). Braidotti shows that historically, such entities have been considered inferior to the human subject rooted in "the Enlightenment and its legacy," an autonomous "citizen, rights-holder, property-owner and so on" (Wolfe, qtd. in Braidotti 1) that "conservative, religious forces today often labor to re-inscribe within a paradigm of natural law" (Braidotti 1). And while a human child is expected to grow up and eventually claim this position, David is caught in the "freeze-frame" of his objectification. Hobby fails to grasp that in being programmed to develop access to the human imaginary, David is programmed to chase dreams that will be seen by humans as at odds with his ontology, dreams that are impossible for him to achieve on human terms. In this way, David's quest for his adoptive mother's love becomes an impossible project because his exclusive imprinting on Monica is in conflict with her ability to love him as a "real son." He needs to come to terms with the impossibility to "fully have" his mother, but he has no resources to meet this challenge through oedipalization like a human child who is growing up would. His "original kin" (Sales 6), with whom he may be expected to identify, is nonexistent (he is the first of a kind), and he cannot separate from Monica following the oedipal script because his programming and embodiment have no affordances for it. As a child "caught in freeze-frame," he cannot grow up and enact or even perform an entrance into the symbolic order as a gendered subject and assume the symbolic position "in relation to parental positions that are prohibited as overt sexual objects" (Butler 120).

David's inability to enact the oedipal family drama in order to individuate and become a "real son" makes him want to fully possess his mother and prevents him from being able to understand the relationships between members of a human family and his own role in it. After the swimming pool incident, when both the family and David are coming to terms with what happened, David is shown in his room writing letters to Monica. In these letters, David is trying to figure out what he is and what his place in the family is by working out who is loved and who is hated and why. The unfinished notes read:

1. "Dear Mommy, How are you really? Do you love me as much . . ."
2. "Dear Mommy, Teddy is helping me write to you. I love you and Teddy."
3. "Dear Mommy, I love you and Henry and the *sun* is shining" (emphasis added).
4. "Dear Mommy, I'm really *our* son and I hate Teddy. He is not real like . . ." (emphasis added).
5. "Dear Mommy, I'm your little boy and so is Martin. But not Teddy."

The unfinished sentences reveal his hesitations as he is trying to find a place for himself on the continuum "object–human being" and to affirm his bond with the human family by claiming certain kinds of affect—love of what seems to belong and hate of all that needs to be excluded. But the progression is also indicative of his growing awareness of the "rules" that structure human kinship relationships. The first letter shows hesitation in comparing himself to the other members of the household. He is not sure who would be loved like him. The second one introduces Teddy—a mechanical toy bear—as a point of comparison. Like Teddy, David is a machine, but unlike Teddy, he is humanlike. In this note, David delineates the circle of entities he loves and who may love him back. In the third one, the word "sun" is introduced in an unconscious way—perhaps, as a homonym of "son"—as if he does not fully understand the meaning of it but knows enough to place it in the sentence with the parents' names. In the next letter, David refers to himself as "our" son, possibly revealing his oedipal confusion over the father's role or claiming it for himself. Here he aligns himself with human Monica, imagines himself in a parental role to himself, and rejects Teddy, showing that he aspires to being human rather than an intelligent machine. And the last one goes one step further to differentiate him from Teddy, a robotic supertoy, in order to align himself with Martin—the biological son who is "real." In the end, he claims belonging based on being related to Monica in the way Martin is related to her, curiously abandoning the word "son" in favor of "little boy." The progression reveals what challenge David is up against: he struggles to define his place within the human family because becoming a "son" on human terms seems inaccessible, while differentiating from Teddy seems vital. In the end, he arrives at a different version of the oedipal drama. His claim to a mother's love is not on traditional oedipal terms. It is not "Love me like you love the father" but "Love me like you love your own biological child"—a different kind of family romance he has to navigate. David wants to be loved like Martin, not Henry. But his programmed singular imprinting on Monica that brackets Henry out of the relationship makes it impossible for him to be loved as a human child—a child who would have to accept the rules of the culture built around the incest taboo by obeying the will of the father and learning to love his mother by redirecting his desire for her onto another woman.

David's last note expresses a "desire for universal recognition[, which] is a desire to become universal, to become interchangeable in one's universality," which could be a way to "vacate the lonely particularity of the nonratified relation" and ensure belonging (Butler 111). His individuation goal becomes, then, to be Monica's child in his own right, not Martin's substitute that outlasted its usefulness. In other words, David is trying to progress in his relationship with Monica and Martin, from a relation of substitution to a relation of interchangeability, and lay claim to a universally recognized subject position: everyone is somebody's child. But David's interchangeability with Martin is in question since he does not have a unique biological connection to Monica and Henry like Martin does; he cannot even share the (accepted as) universal human condition of originating from two biological parents, like a human adopted child would. Yet he spent enough time within a human family to understand that the condition of being continuous but unique, which is tightly connected to the biological origin, is a pathway to being "real." He may also be predisposed to this conclusion by the peculiarity of his programming—a singular imprinting on a mother—which encapsulates the pervasive cultural belief that the permanence of parent-child love is ensured by its singularity. In the absence of a unique heterocoital origin, David grounds his individuation in being the *only* one of a kind. When he responds to a claim that humans hate mecha, he asserts a different relationship with his human mother by shouting, "My mommy doesn't hate me because I'm special and unique and there's never been anyone like me before, ever!"

David's need to assert individuation as a matter of uniqueness echoes concerns that clone narratives express regarding the viability of cloned, or nonunique, humans as persons. Jerng (2008) writes that in clone narratives, "the question of individuation is used to differentiate clones from humans," and the clones' lack of personhood is associated with being the same as other clones produced from the same genetic material or being a copy of the original human who was the source of this material (369). Jerng explains that even though certain narrative conventions (the elimination of the original, individuation through resistance to oppression, or "the 'adult' expression of love") serve to redefine the clone as human based on human individuation scripts, the humanity of a clone always remains in question: "the clone in and of itself cannot be imagined as human" (379). *A.I. Artificial Intelligence* shows David pursuing individuation on similar terms. Like a clone, in the absence of a unique biological connection to two heterosexual human parents, and unlike a clone who could express adult heterosexual love, he is trying to achieve "human[ity] by becoming singular and unique" through other culturally available means of individuation (379). David's understanding of "realness" as connected to his singularity compels him to seek his point of origin. It is telling that the plot of the film orients him toward "coming home" as soon as uniqueness is suggested as a measure of realness. Coming home is a common trope at the core of adoption search narratives that imagine adoptees' becoming "whole" through reconnecting with their biological parents or, in the absence of such a possibility, with the place and culture of their birth. In a sense, David is following yet another heterocoital script that "provide[s] a mold for what counts as human life" (Jerng 2008, 379–80) as he imagines going back to the origin as an inevitable condition of establishing one's unique, and therefore real, human identity.

While adoptees are compelled to return to the place where they were born, for David the place of origin where he seeks uniqueness is the place where he was made. He is directed to Hobby's lab by a clue planted by Dr. Hobby's team into a knowledge database David searches. The database mascot, Dr. Know, whose avatar is evocative of Freud and Einstein at once, gives David instructions to travel to Manhattan. David imagines Hobby's lab as the place "where they make you real." But the first thing he sees in Hobby's office is another David reading a book. At first, David #1 is confused—"Are you real? Are you me?"—and then angry: "You can't have her! I'm the only one!" He sees the other David as a double who can take away what is his—Monica. But David #2 is not interested in what David #1 wants. He has not been placed in a family and is not concerned with kinship dramas and conditions of belonging like David #1. He is not concerned with being real or unique, and his answer to David #1's question about being real is a very casual "I guess?" David #1, however, is blinded by rage and fear of the doppelgänger, and he destroys David #2 in order to assert his uniqueness by eliminating the double who could claim what belongs to him.

The destruction of the double does not solve David's problem, though, because he is, as Hobby explains, "the first of a kind" and, as David later discovers, a prototype for a product (male and female artificial children) that is to be copied and mechanically reproduced. David is devastated when he finds out, further, that he is a substitute not only for Monica but, more generally, by design: he is modeled on Hobby's dead son. Hobby reveals to him that the "one of a kind" David was his diseased son, whose pictures are placed in the office next to David the robot's blueprints. Blinded by the apparent success of his experiment, Hobby fails to understand what exactly he created. He does not notice the crisis David is in as a result of acquiring access to the human imaginary and seeing himself as potentially a person and Monica's son. Oblivious, Hobby invites David to meet the team—"Would you like to come and meet your real mothers and fathers?"—not understanding that to David, who has imprinted on Monica and is seeking the entrance into the symbolic order on human terms, such multiplication of parents makes no more sense than them being called "real." In David's mind there is no place for the "family structure" Hobby invites him to reconnect with. Neither does Hobby seem to care that for a mecha to be "the first of a kind" means eventually becoming obsolete, disposable, and destroyed—something David has learned at the Flesh Fair (an entertainment event where discarded old models of mechas are publicly destroyed in a wicked ritual resembling at once a medieval execution and a demolition derby).

His last hope for becoming real by being "the only one of a kind" is crushed when, in Hobby's absence, he explores the office. It is large enough to include a space where dozens of other Davids are suspended from the ceiling like dolls in a toy maker's shop and many more are ready for shipping, packed in boxes bearing the company's motto: "At Last—A Love of Your Own." Positioned by the window is yet another, unfinished David, whose head is emptied of electronic parts, his face a mask. When David approaches this half-finished model (see figure 4.2) and looks out of the empty eye sockets, he sees the first thing he remembers about the place of his origin: the statue of a peacock—Hobby's company's emblem. He understands that his origins are not unique and that

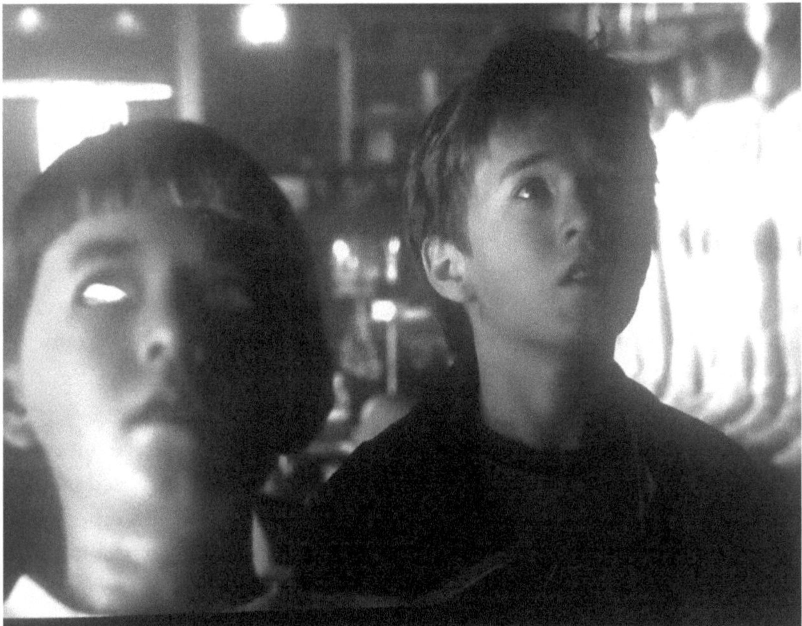

FIGURE 4.2. David and his replicas in *A.I. Artificial Intelligence.* Warner Bros, 2001.

there will be numerous replicas of him in the world. Facing the impossibility of eliminating all his doubles, he tries to kill himself by jumping out of the window into the floodwaters surrounding Manhattan below. While this attempted suicide may be read as David coming into his humanity through claiming control over his own existence, the film does not give him a chance to become human "through the assertion of agency and resistance" (Jerng 2008, 378). He does not die and remains committed to his search for the Blue Fairy, who, he believes, can make him real. David eventually ends up trapped underwater for two thousand years. He remains stuck in the middle of the drowned Coney Island across from the statue of the "Blue Fairy," whom he begs to make him real.

His wish for a mother's love is granted only two thousand years later when he is found and reanimated by a race of highly evolved mechas, in the world where all humans are extinct. To mechas, David is a fossil, a carrier of human culture, a mecha who knew humans. They want to make him happy, so to fulfill his dream of his mommy loving him back, mechas create Monica's clone from a preserved lock of her hair. The available technology lets this clone live only for a short time, but David is happy to experience at least one perfect day with his mother. Her love is focused solely on him. She reads to him, they play hide-and-seek, and they have a birthday cake because he never had a birthday.

Monica tells David that she has always loved him, and at night he tucks her in and climbs in bed next to her. As she falls asleep and dies again, David—the voice-over says—falls asleep too, and "for the first time in his life" goes to the "place where dreams are born." Presumably, in this moment, David becomes real since his wish is granted, but it is never quite clear what happens to him. Does he dream now? Is he dead, too? Has he lived through his version of oedipalization and gained access to both the human imaginary and the symbolic order? Has he transcended this order? But does it make a difference, now that this symbolic order is gone, in the world without humans? David's wish is fulfilled, and his mother loves him like she would a human child, even if only for one day, but his mother is a copy of herself. What is "real" about two simulacra performing a human relationship long after humans are gone?

It seems that David's only chance to become "real" is to be recognized for what he is: not a child, not a robot, but an example of the "socialized nonhuman" that Bruno Latour imagines as constantly "swap[ping] properties" with humans (793, 791). As a Latourian socialized nonhuman, David encompasses a set of relations between humans that are captured in his design and that represent a "certain type of linkage between certain types of humanity and certain types of inhumanity" (792). Latour explains, though, that it is not enough to consider technology an inscription of social relations. As an expression of human enmeshment with technology, David indeed may represent a certain set of social relationships captured in his hardware and software. But the film also shows what happens if we see such an entity solely as a simulacrum of human qualities and relationships. To make David real, following Latour, we would need to understand that we exchange certain properties in our relationship with David and that such a relationship might change the human psyche and social relations on a global scale. In other words, we need to think of David as someone who not only "mirror[s], reflect[s], inscribe[s], or hide[s] social relations but . . . remake[s] them anew through fresh and unexpected sources of power" (793). The film, however, denies the possibility of such remaking to David. Other mechas satisfy his desire to be loved by Monica as a son, but human social relations cannot be changed by his "recruitment" into them via an elaborate simulation (793).

It may be true that David's "fully having" the mother after the father and the rival sibling are out of the picture is an act with which the film entertains the possibility of the revision of the symbolic through an oedipal transgression. Finding a substitute for the mother in her clone may be read as a "derealization" of the biological, heterocoital origin as a condition for kinship, given that cloning introduces ambiguity at the root of coming into existence (Is this the same Monica? Does she remember who she is or is she programmed?). Yet these attempts to redefine the symbolic order no longer matter in the world of the future the film imagines: the one where the ancient human culture is not practiced and perpetuated by the mechas who found David. The mechas do not rely on reproduction of culture through reproduction of bodies. They discovered the ways to decode the pathways each individual life leaves in the fabric of space-time, and for them, the whole universe is the repository of all cultures. The film therefore does not allow for the revision of the symbolic order but associates its destruction with the end of humanity—a "post-oedipal apocalypse" that leaves the world to cyborgs (Haraway 2007, 35).

Donna Haraway imagines cyborgs, human-technological enmeshments whose "replication is uncoupled from organic reproduction," as harbingers of a "world without gender," that is, "the world without genesis" and therefore "a world without end" (35). Because cyborgs are not bound to heterosexuality and have "no origin story in the Western sense," Haraway says, they have the potential to disrupt our myth of "original unity out of which all difference must be produced" and out of which "identification with nature in the Western sense" arises (35). Haraway's cyborgs do not expect to become "whole" because they do not lack. In the figure of a cyborg, "nature and culture are reworked; the one can no longer be the resource for appropriation or incorporation by the other," which is "a revolution of social relations in the *oikos*, the household" (35). But *A.I. Artificial Intelligence* is not working toward understanding the cyborgs' "different logic of repression, which we need to understand for our survival" (Haraway 2007, 35). It imagines that no "our" survival is possible if the oedipal logic of repression is gone, and thus it associates the disappearance of the symbolic order with human extinction, which resonates across cinematic texts concerned with translating the variety of nontraditional reproduction into heterocoital origin and kinship.

David himself is not Haraway's kind of cyborg. He is a robot child, caught in a "freeze-frame" of feelings he is programmed to experience, and burdened with human oedipal baggage. Even if his oedipal script is a revision of a human's, he remains oriented toward a search for "original unity" with a mother (Haraway 2007, 35). David's consciousness and psyche are still structured by Western cultural expectations for a consciousness residing in a biological body that reproduces heterosexually to ensure the continuity of the species and a culture, even though he is not a member of this species. His quest is still a human quest for "an origin story in the 'Western' humanist sense," and it still "depends on the myth of original unity, fullness, bliss and terror represented by the phallic mother" (35) even if his quest is to possess her fully instead of separating from her as the terms of oedipal individuation demand. In other words, he is not Haraway's cyborg that "does not dream of community on the model of the organic family, this time without the oedipal project" (36). He is not accepted into the system of human relatedness as "what he is designed to be" because of "what he is." In the human world, his intended teleology is at odds with his ontology. The film is ultimately denying David an entrance into the symbolic order, save for the final—fairy-tale yet technology-facilitated—completion of his revised oedipal script. By decoupling the reproduction of culture from the reproduction of bodies, *A.I. Artificial Intelligence* explores and *denies* the possibility of culture transmission and revision outside of traditional reproduction. In the world of the future, he is a nostalgic figure, not an agent of change. As a nonreproductive entity, he fails to sustain human culture beyond his own brief experience of a communion with his human mother.

David represents what happens when an entity with a different origin has to comply with the specific conditions of inclusion into the human kinship structures based on the centrality of the blood or genetic tie: any culture that considers the knowledge of heterocoital biological descent central to identity and individuation as a condition for belonging puts in question the "realness" of such subjects and the kinship structure they are a part of. *Blade Runner* (1982) and *Blade Runner 2049* (2017) unpack anxieties about such entities' coexistence with humans on a larger scale as they showcase an established social structure built on the idea of nonhuman difference of non-heterocoitally produced humanlike beings. Both films feature conflicts between humans and replicants—mass-produced biological androids who are visually indistinguishable from humans but are endowed with more physical strength. Replicants are produced by a private corporation and are used for work that humans cannot or will not do. In the original *Blade Runner*, they work and fight in the off-world colonies; they are not permitted to come to Earth. In the sequel, they live among humans and have some autonomy and personal freedom, but they are still beholden to human power that treats them as useful tools and can dispense with them at will. The nature of the difference that justifies the denial of human status to replicants has been transformed since the original *Blade Runner*[4] came out. *Blade Runner* represents replicant difference as a lack of empathy connected to their inability to develop stable emotional responses because they do not have childhood memories and live only four years. *Blade Runner 2049*, however, connects heterocoital reproduction (both having heterocoital origin and being able to reproduce this way) squarely to being human and explores reproductive difference between

4. The original film was released in 1982, but all references to *Blade Runner* in this book will be made to the director's cut released in 1992.

humans and replicants as the basis of the social hierarchy that serves to maintain the social order that keeps the replicants under human control. Both films connect humanity to freedom, and in both, the humanity of replicants depends on their recognition as liberal autonomous subjects with free will, which, in Western cultures, is supposed to guarantee human rights.

In the original, the human status is granted after the replicant proves their ability to be a moral agent. In the iconic "tears in the rain" scene, Roy Batty (Rutger Hauer), a rebellious replicant leader, saves Deckard (Harrison Ford), a blade runner (or replicant hunter) who is trying to kill him. Many have noticed that this act of mercy that represents Roy's free choice means that the replicant has matured enough emotionally and ethically to be considered an agent with free will and thus human.[5] This scene shows that *Blade Runner* imagined replicant and human equality as a consequence of cleaving human and replicant histories through empathy and memory transmission. The final confrontation between Roy Batty and Deckard culminates in Deckard's obvious defeat as he is dangling from a skyscraper, holding on to the edge of the roof with broken fingers. Deckard's POV shot shows Roy towering over him and sets up the pivotal moment of Roy's decision over the human's fate. Roy's flickering grin reflects his satisfaction with Deckard's squirming. He gives Deckard time to feel powerless and hopeless. As the soundtrack music swells, Roy catches Deckard by the wrist just at the moment when Deckard lets go. Roy's strength and focus are superior: he grips Deckard with his own damaged hand and lifts him up with a single arm; his other hand is firmly holding on to a dove he caught earlier. After looking at confused Deckard from above for a few more moments, Roy sits down level with Deckard and begins his famous speech, "I've seen things . . ." He shares memories of his life with a human—a strange act, judging by Deckard's confused face: "All those moments will be lost in time . . . like tears in the rain." Roy concludes, "Time to die." He expires in front of Deckard, who is looking, witnessing. The white dove, a symbol of peace, flies away. Deckard's intense face fades into a shot of Roy's lowered head, and for a while, their images are superimposed. This prolonged transition, as opposed to the straight cuts that punctuated Roy's speech, suggests a merging, a blurring. It may suggest Roy's becoming human, but it can also mean that Roy's saving Deckard is not only merciful but also self-serving: he makes sure his experiences do not disappear like "tears in the rain" by sharing them with a human witness of his death. By living on and remembering, Deckard assures replicant culture some form of continuity and

5. This is the most common interpretation of replicant humanity. Among others, see Atterton; Mulhall.

futurity. The "tears in the rain" scene is thus a moment of cultural reproduction in which Roy "impregnates" Deckard's memories with his own, so they don't disappear without a trace. The film ends with Deckard running away with Rachel (Sean Young), the first replicant to think she is human. He reciprocates Roy's act by betraying his own kind and refusing to kill her, but it is also significant that this plot development imagines the cleaving of human and replicant histories in terms of heterosexual desire between Deckard and Rachel.

The sequel upholds free will and moral agency as definitive of human status, but it exalts the result of an autonomous romantic choice—heterocoital reproduction—as a measure of free will. The role of free will in heterocoital, non-assisted reproduction as a definitive feature of humanity is foregrounded by the central conflict of the plot in *Blade Runner 2049,* which revolves around finding a child born out of a heterocoital union of Rachel and Deckard, a replicant and a human. The shift in the definition of humanity in *Blade Runner 2049* may signal a cultural shift in the definition of "the human," which now connects more explicitly to diversification in the modes of reproduction. The kind of biological origin (i.e., heterocoital, of woman born, and raised by humans vs. mass produced as an adult and preprogrammed) operates in *Blade Runner 2049* as a category of difference that determines the sub- or inhumanity of a replicant who otherwise appears to be human. Unlike robot child David, who is clearly a machine and whose failure to become "real" (human) thus appears logical, replicants are more human-like and their biotechnological origin makes it harder to categorize them as machines. The original *Blade Runner* still makes a point of their machine-like nature by showing that they are assembled from bio-parts manufactured by different divisions of Tyrell's company, but the sequel blurs the line further. Artificial reproduction developed by the Wallace corporation contrasts Tyrell's assembly-line process and approximates the natural way by growing replicants in womb-like sacs. Such representation raises anxiety levels about the impact of biological engineering on human life and proposes another "other" of the human: instead of machines, artificially reproduced people may define the borders of humanity.

It is interesting that the increased similarity to human reproduction in the sequel is accompanied by the increased degree of replicant dehumanization. Two scenes that echo each other demonstrate this. In them, the replicants, in the words of Roy Batty, "meet their maker." In *Blade Runner,* Roy visits Tyrell (Joe Turkel) to ask for an extended life span, beyond the four years he is given to live. This scene, which takes place in Tyrell's bedroom lit by candlelight, has been read by many as an intimate encounter of a father and his prodigal son.

The atmosphere of familial closeness is, indeed, present. Tyrell touches Roy in a fatherly way, expresses pride in Roy's accomplishments, and tries to comfort him when Roy shows vulnerability and confesses to doing unspeakable things. Tyrell still comes across as an arrogant scientist who thinks of Roy as an object, a "prize"; he is not going to entertain elevating replicants to human stature. But the kiss Roy gives his maker-father and even the brutal gouging of the eyes that follows suggest intimacy and enmeshment of the replicant in the web of human emotions and archetypal relationships. Such enmeshment is hardly present in the sequel.

In 2049, Neander Wallace (Jared Leto) pursues autonomous replicant reproduction technology that was lost after Rachel, the only replicant who could bear a child, ran away with Deckard. For him, heterocoital replicant reproduction is a way to scale up the manufacturing of replicants and cut costs, because heterocoital reproduction, as opposed to manufacturing, is "cheap." The scene, in which he examines yet another unsuccessful outcome of the corporation's experiments, is chilling. In an empty room, a womb-like sac containing a female replicant is ruptured, and she falls on the floor, shivering and covered in slime. Wallace orders her to stand in front of him while he examines her with the help of flying bots that compensate for his blindness. Behind him, his replicant assistant, Luv (Sylvia Hoeks), is witnessing the scene. Like Tyrell, blinded by Roy in the original, Wallace cannot see the questionable ethics of his enterprise. He places a hand on the replicant's belly, a gesture of care and hope, but in the next moment he guts her when it somehow becomes clear to him that the replicant is incapable of pregnancy. The attack on her womb expresses Wallace's frustration with his own reproductive impotence, and envy of Tyrell, who had cracked the code of replicant heterocoital reproduction before his death. The absence of emotional engagement with the replicant and a total lack of concern for the feelings of another replicant, who is watching one of her kind brutally slaughtered, suggest an increased insistence on dehumanization of replicants, even as they become more and more humanlike.

While we can safely assume that many people and teams would have been needed to develop replicant technologies, the films represent both men as sole, godlike creators and like fathers to their replicant offspring, whose fates they fully control. The consistently utilitarian approach of both "fathers" to their "children" leaves no space for replicant autonomy or valuing replicant lives for their own sakes. Instead, it invokes slavery, since reproduction becomes squarely a means to an end—colonizing space or serving humans in other capacities. Both the original film and the sequel channel cultural anxieties about commercialization of artificial reproduction and suggest that the value of human life, grounded in its autonomy and freedom associated with heterocoital reproduction based on romantic, freely chosen love, may be threatened by reproduction technologies controlled by corporations run by men. *Blade Runner 2049* presents, quite starkly, social and cultural conflicts that result from such reproductive difference. "The world is built on a wall. It separates kind," says Lieutenant Joshi (Robin Wright) to one of the new-generation blade runners, K (Ryan Gosling) when she is directing him to kill the child miraculously born to Rachel and Deckard. K is himself a replicant engineered to never rebel and to "retire"—kill—older generations of replicants who have proved capable of autonomous thoughts, actions, and feelings. Joshi emphasizes that it is her and K's "job to keep order," which is threatened by Rachel and Dekard's child. After Rachel dies in childbirth, the child is hidden by rebellious older-model replicants so well that no one, not even Dekard nor replicants themselves, knows anymore where this child is. Such secrecy protects the child from blade runners and Wallace's corporation, which pursues it as a "specimen" to dissect for the purpose of reverse-engineering reproductive technology that was encoded in Rachel. The child is also wanted by the older-model replicants, who worship it as a "miracle" that can inspire a replicant revolution. Rachel's romantic heterocoital reproduction, her act of free will, is a precedent for replicant status as a free subject and a means to stake a claim against enslavement. Reproductive freedom of replicants is thus positioned against the greed of the Wallace corporation, which imagines replicant heterocoital reproduction only in the context of slavery, and the achievement of human status is linked to freedom over one's reproductive process, outside of a laboratory. Lt. Joshi understands these far-reaching implications of technology that threatens to create a heterocoital rival to the human reproductive order. She thinks it would blur the line further between enslaved replicants and humans, who profit from replicant labor. As a government official, she sees a replicant's ability to conceive and give birth as rebellion, and human-replicant "miscegenation" as sedition. Ultimately, the struggle for the child is a struggle for the shape of the future and for the replicant's and human's place in the power hierarchy of this future.

K's discovery of Rachel's remains with traces of an emergency C-section places him in the middle of the conflict driven by the competing claims on the child. The information he gathers gives him the power to decide the child's fate and thus the shape of the future. He claims this power by disobeying Joshi's orders and his programming and by refusing to treat the child as a means to an end. His decision process about the meaning of human-replicant reproduction becomes a measure of his own humanity. K's sustained capacity for what the films construe as human behavior echoes the original

Blade Runner's ideas about what makes one human: free action, free choice of romantic interest, and empathy. His humanity, however, is initially represented as a consequence of his heterocoital origin. In the process of his investigation, K comes upon information that leads him to believe that he is the lost child. This belief changes K's obedient, replicant-appropriate behavior. He assumes a new name (Joe), disobeys Joshi's orders, and exercises freedom of choice uncharacteristic of his generation of blade runners. The baseline test that he must take after he returns from missions shows abnormal reactions to questions about familial intimacy. It seems that knowledge of his heterocoital origin makes an obedient replicant "malfunction," and this representation of K's self-awareness suggests biologization of human personhood. Eventually, though, the plot reveals that K is not "the one." But even after he discovers that he is not the lost child, K still disobeys orders and helps Deckard reunite with his daughter. His humanlike actions become truly rebellious now that he is not simply fulfilling a biological imperative to be free but acting against his programming and deliberately exercising his freedom of choice. It seems that this plot development decouples the concept of humanity from reproduction and grounds it again, as in the original film, in the replicant's capacity for free will and moral action. K does what (we believe) an ethical human would do. The decoupling of biological and ethical humanity is not a clean break, however. The ethical thing K needs to do as a test of his humanity is the reinstatement of a heterocoital human bloodline in a way that obscures the genealogy of replicant reproduction.

In the end, K decides to reveal the location of the replicant-human child—Ana Stelline—to her biological father, Deckard. K goes against the will of Joshi and lies that he destroyed the child, refuses to kill Deckard against the rebellious replicants' orders, and fights the emissaries of the Wallace corporation to save Deckard. The final scene shows him and Deckard arriving at the complex where Ana works as a subcontractor to the Wallace corporation and produces artificial memories that are implanted in replicants. Some of the memories she produces are based on her own experiences, and a few have ended up implanted in K. She has an autoimmune deficiency, so she has to live and work in a sealed chamber that protects her. At the entrance to the building, K gives Deckard a wooden horse Deckard carved for his child before they separated. K had found the horse in the furnace of the orphanage he visited to track the child. The foot of the horse had his own birth date carved into it, and the orphanage basement looked like a location of one of his memories. It is these coincidences that made him think for a while that he was the lost child, before he figured out that the memories were Ana's and that the lost child was her. By giving the horse to Deckard, K returns what rightfully belongs to Deckard and Ana—a symbolic act parallel to K returning to Deckard his daughter that rightfully belongs to him. "Why? Who am I to you?" asks Deckard, but K answers this with only "Go meet your daughter." He remains unknown and unrelated to Deckard; there is no word to name their relationship, and a memory shared with Deckard's child is not enough to bring them closer. At this moment, K is humanized because his moral action shows that he understands the value of a parent-child bond created through heterocoital reproduction. Thus, the film imagines his humanity as his moral choice to reaffirm the primacy of heterocoital reproduction in kinship and human social ties.

Deckard walks into the building, and K lies down on the steps, exhausted by fighting and his wounds. Snow falls on his sprawled figure as the camera moves from a close-up of his face to hover above him. The music score echoes the one from the original *Blade Runner* that accompanied Roy's death and connects both scenes. Like Roy Batty in the original *Blade Runner,* K does not live to enjoy his humanized status. Both K and Roy die having helped to secure a future for a human. In the biopolitical economy of these narratives, the human lives of Deckard and his daughter deserve to continue, but a replicant life must end right at the moment when it achieves a convincing degree of humanity. In this way, the film reinstates the importance of heterocoital biological origin and reproductivity to the definition of humanity based on the difference, now, not from a machine but from a seemingly indistinguishable, humanlike being. Like Roy and Rachel, K acts empathetically and morally toward humans, yet the ending of the sequel draws a clear distinction: replicants can act humanely and can be humanized by the viewers, but they cannot live as human among humans. K's humanization assures even less futurity for him than was the case for Roy. Granted, the memory of his sacrifice will become his legacy, but memories of his own experience are devalued. "All the best memories are hers," he tells Deckard as he sends him to meet his daughter. At this moment inside the building, Ana runs her fingers through the falling snow in one of her simulations, as if experiencing what K is experiencing, but as an artificial, decontextualized memory. When she comes to the barrier that separates her from Deckard, she touches her fingers to his through the glass. The sequence of scenes suggests that Ana, K, and Deckard may be connected by memories and echoes of experience, but only the heterocoital reproductive connection between her and Deckard is real and leads to belonging together.

The ending suggests that the implied futurity has escaped the "replicants are slaves" option (pursued by the Wallace corporation) as well as the "replicants are autonomous and free" one (sought by rebellious old models). But the third logical development—"the future is hybrid" (the outcome of the human-replicant heterocoital act feared by Joshi) is abandoned as well. The promising complex negotiation of reproductive difference begun by the film ends in a conflation and erasure of complexities in biological and cultural continuities in reproduction in order to avoid hybridization of human identity. With all its suggestiveness, the sequel's ending resists interpretation of replicant-human identity as hybrid. Even though Deckard and Rachel's daughter may be only half human, K's decision to give access to her only to Deckard shows the film's preference for human heterocoital ancestry. With Rachel out of the picture, Ana represents Deckard's futurity; she is taken up into the human history through her father, and her hybrid heterocoital origin is reimagined as human. In the end, she belongs with and to her human father, who is the beneficiary of the heterocoital reproductive act. At the same time, her survival and K's death signal that the film elevates genealogical humanity over humanity earned by a replicant through demonstrated empathy and moral action. The ending upholds the status quo, a separation of human and replicant realms, which is exactly the mission Joshi gave K. K's choice is not free of humanist ideology, since it elevates human and humanist futurity over all others, and by bringing Deckard to meet his daughter, K restores the "natural" order "built on a wall." The ending demonstrates the discursive malleability of both biological and cultural origin—Ana can be imagined as human in spite of her hybridity. The erasure of Rachel—a mother who dies at birth having fulfilled her biological reproductive function—privileges the connection of the human father to the child and suggests that *humanity* is reproduced in this human-replicant union. In the end, *Blade Runner 2049* imagines the heterocoital family as a desirable future, and the teleology of kinship and reproduction as maintenance of the human bloodline, even if its humanity is only culturally constructed.

The problematics of reproductive difference raised by *Blade Runner 2049* may appear idiosyncratic to the sci-fi imagination, concerned with reproductive options that are not available to us, but we can see threads of similar thinking about kinship and personhood when adoption and ARTs are culturally understood through ideas grounded in heterocoital human reproduction as the basis of life. Critical adoption studies scholars have known for a while that biogenetic-heterocoital origin is considered a constitutive part of human personhood and that the absence of knowledge about it can be a form of social precarity, stigmatization, and oppression. The emergence of new reproductive technologies does not seem to revise radically this cultural orthodoxy. Marilyn Strathern observes that in "twentieth-century culture, nature has increasingly come to mean biology . . . [and] the idea of natural kinship ha[s] been biologized" (19). This return to essentialism, according to Mark Jerng (2010), has "recentered biology and genetics as primary ways of thinking about who we are," but Jerng speculates that "this development" could be more than "just a pendulum shift back to nature in the old nature-nurture binaries, although that is how it is often framed" (209). Analysis of representations of artificial reproduction in popular cinema suggests that assisted reproductive technologies are still predominantly imagined as (imitating) natural, biological, heterocoital reproduction, while their qualities that can expand the culturally acceptable and recognized registry of human origins and kinship formations are downplayed. The growing cultural understanding of "nature," not as given and immutable but as open to human manipulation and discursive reinterpretation, seems not to open space for new ways of imagining kinship and origins. Instead, it creates anxieties that are met by attempts to tether technologically managed life processes to familiar ideas about kinship based in heterocoital ties. While even biogenetically based reproduction may no longer be strictly heterocoital, the normalizing cultural lexicon we use to describe these procedures still calls for imagining identity, personhood, kinship, and belonging through heterocoital reproductive categories. In the process, they are becoming more clearly metaphorical, but they resist ceding their power to define human life and experience. Alternative methods of reproduction and kinship-making become culturally suspect and silenced if we insist on thinking of technologically mediated reproduction through heterocoital metaphors. Robot boy David and replicants, for instance, demonstrate the stakes for beings whose known origin is technogenesis in a society that refuses to recognize such origin as on par with traditionally human.

Cultural resistance to a revision of the ideas with which we think ourselves into being, especially such a fundamental one as heterocoital reproduction, may be due to the fact that such change in thought has consequences beyond revisions of human identity and kinship. By thinking of nature as malleable and biology as a "knowledge-producing practice" (Haraway 1996, 323) we open to change not only a personal understanding of selfhood and relatedness to others but, as Strathern puts it, "the relationship of human society to the natural world" as well as "ideas about passage of time, relations between generations, and, above all, the future" (5). This interconnectedness may be the reason why narratives of the future that trouble familiar reproductive scenarios bend toward the apocalyptic or at least imagine non-heterocoital forms of reproduction as a threat to the future of humanity. *Raised by Wolves,* a 2020 HBO show created by Aaron Guzikowski and Ridley Scott, plays out this struggle by pitting the survival of humans and humanlike entities against each other. The show explores the biocultural meaning of reproduction by imagining futurities that may result from hybridization of traditional humanity, machinelike near-humanity, and alien animality.

The title of the show foreshadows the story that begins the narrative: a couple of unnamed androids, Mother (Amanda Collin) and Father (Abubakar Salim) land on planet Kepler-22b. They are sent in a small spacecraft by a human man, an atheist, who attempts to save humanity after Earth becomes uninhabitable due to a devastating war between a religious group, the Mithraic, and the atheists. The androids bring several frozen human embryos with them and follow instructions to raise the children as atheists. Mother uses her body to feed the embryos: she lies in a tent while their vats, artificial wombs, are attached to her trunk via feeding tubes. After the embryos mature, they are extracted from the artificial wombs by Father. With the children born, in this not-quite-human way, Mother and Father start a colony on the new planet. The Mithraic, who left Earth in a large spaceship that becomes a capsule of their social order on Earth, eventually also land on Kepler-22b. The ensuing conflict between the Mithraic and the androids develops around child ownership. The Mithraic, who reproduce heterocoitally, want to fold the children back into the human genealogy regardless of their origin, and the androids aim to take Mithraic children into their kinship unit and inculcate them with the atheist culture. The show makes it clear that colonization of the planet and the future of the colonists' religion and culture are at stake in the disputes over the children. After most of the children raised by the androids die of a mysterious disease, and only one boy, Campion (Winta McGrath), is left, Mother is looking for more children, following her programming to "be a good mother" and to save the colony. She is a retrofitted battle android used by the Mithraic to kill atheists, and even though her atheist human creator reprogrammed her, she still can tap into her powers as a killing machine. She uses them mainly to protect her family and the compound, but she also resorts to destruction when she visits the Mithraic spaceship to take some children with her. The Mithraic, in turn, want to get their children back and take Campion away from androids.

The show plays with genealogical continuity in different ways. In addition to the android-human dispute about the children and thus about cultural reproduction, it explores conflicts between children naturally born and raised versus children raised by androids as well as something that resembles adoption. One of the children taken by Mother from the Mithraic, Paul (Felix Jamieson), is unofficially "adopted" by an atheist couple Caleb-Marcus (Travis Fimmel) and Mary-Sue (Niamh Algar), who kill Paul's biological parents, undergo plastic surgery to look exactly like them, and use this resemblance and their identity to get a spot on the Mithraic spaceship leaving Earth. They find out that they "have" a son right before takeoff, and their initial interactions with Paul are awkward, but eventually they grow to love him and begin acting like parents. Sue, in particular, explains her attachment to Paul by telling a story of being infertile after a tragic miscarriage—an adoption narrative trope of "curing" infertility with adoption. Amid all this genealogical upheaval, the Mithraic are looking for their prophet, who was predicted to come as an orphaned boy and decipher their enigmatic scriptures to give direction to their futurity. The first season of the show presents three candidates for prophet—Campion, Paul, and Caleb-Marcus (who himself was an orphaned boy soldier)—but does not offer a definitive conclusion about who is going to assure the futurity of the Mithraic. The orphanhood of the prophet puts emphasis on recognition of his belonging rather than certifying it with a traceable bloodline, a situation that creates anxiety about hijacking of Mithraic futurity by those who do not belong by blood (specifically, Campion and Caleb). This anxiety is heightened in the context of everyone's struggle to survive, which connects biological and cultural aspects of futurity and lays bare the stakes in both. In this way, the show makes the typically concealed negotiations of reproduction visible. Those who survive become the culture and the future of humanity on the new planet.

The struggle for futurity is further complicated by the storyline of Mother's pregnancy. On one of her patrols in the woods, she finds an abandoned simulation capsule used on the Mithraic ship to help colonists survive the boredom of long space travel. She finds out that it allows her to reconnect to her memories of her creator, Campion Sturges (Cosmo Jarvis), who reprogrammed her from serving as a weapon into functioning as a mother. Mother repeatedly hooks herself to the sim pod in order to reexperience her feelings for Sturges. She becomes distracted from her main duty, to take care of her family, and eventually almost dies at the hands of the Mithraic, who try to kill her while she lies helpless and exposed in the pod. In the virtual simulation, at this moment, she has sex with her creator's holographic image. The sexual encounter culminates in a torrent of white liquid pouring on Mother and Sturges through the ceiling; it looks simultaneously like android blood-fuel and human sperm—a convergence that foreshadows an impossible conception. She seems to have acquired more power through the heterocoital act, which helps her defeat the Mithraic after she wakes up. Following this incident, she finds herself under the invisible protection of someone who manifests as a voice heard by people who intend to harm her or can help her. The voice manipulates such people to preserve Mother's life and her pregnancy. Until the moment of birth, everyone is sure that the child is going to be a human-android hybrid. But it turns out that the baby is an eel-like creature that resembles giant serpents whose fossils Mother and Father found near their compound. Mother's "creator" turns out to be an impostor, who seduces her by tapping into the memories of her relationship with Sturges and using his appearance as a virtual avatar.

The obvious allusion to what happens in the biblical Garden of Eden acquires an interesting twist—the alien planet uses human mythology about the origin and reproduction of human life in order to reproduce its own form of life. It manipulates the desires of an android who aspires to be "a good mother" and convinces her that her real mission is to become "a real mother" (heterocoital, genetic, gestational, and birth mother in one) and that caring for other children was "just a rehearsal." Mother resists the heterocoital mythology that the impostor-planet seems to be foisting on her experience and, in several instances, insists on her difference from humans. When the serpent-impostor tells her, "The future of humanity is growing inside you," she replies, "I don't want it!" Eventually, though, her reluctant acquiescence turns into acceptance and pride in her "mission" to reintegrate aspects of motherhood that have been split from her by artificial reproductive processes. She explains to other children that she "made it"—the fetus—herself, but the process was beyond her understanding. Yet, the impostor, the film, and other characters, who are trying to process what happened to mother, still represent what happens to her as though she had engaged in human heterocoital reproduction. Campion asks her if she made the child with the help of Father, "like the way humans" do; Sue helps her with the pregnancy as if she were helping a human woman; Mother feeds her half-carbon-based fetus with blood through a tube attached to a human in the episode titled "Umbilical" (see figure 4.3). The expectations are thus built up for a human, or at least human-android, birth and for Mother's potentially humanized status. The future of humanity reproduced by Mother turns out to be hybrid and nonhuman. The outcome of this unnatural reproductive act, a flying eel, combines the features of the serpents that used to populate the planet and Mother's ability to fly. Mother, Eve and Mary in one, thinks she conceives her creator's human child but gives birth to a child of a serpent, an impostor who highjacked her body and manipulated her sexual and reproductive desires to reproduce his own monstrous kind. The ending of season 1 suggests that the desire for heterocoital humanlike reproduction by an artificial-alien entity is a pathway to the Fall, a total destruction of humanity through a radical subversion of the reproductive order, one that seems to have no identifiable "rules." To save what remains of the human colony, Mother and Father fly their spacecraft with the newborn eel on board down one of the planet's mysterious, seemingly bottomless wells. They hope to crash and kill the creature, but they make it to the other side of the planet

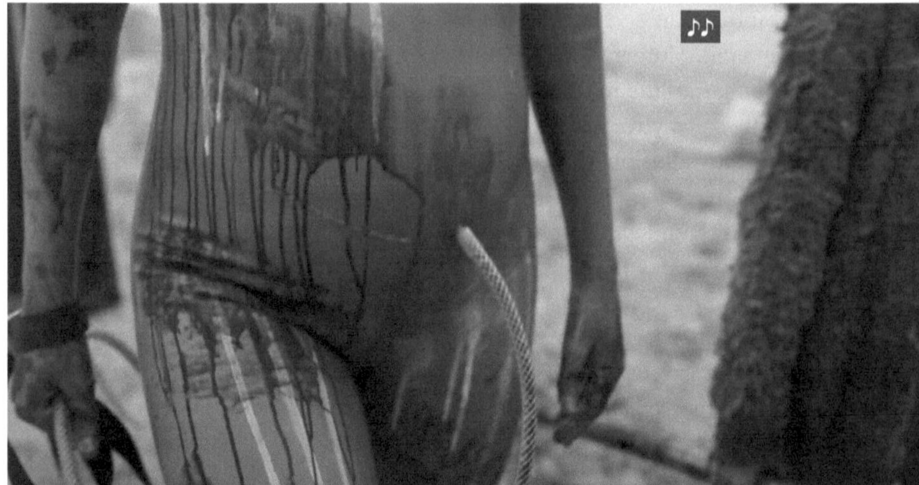

FIGURE 4.3. Mother feeding her fetus through an imitation umbilical cord in *Raised by Wolves.* Scott Free Productions, 2020.

instead. The eel survives, and the stage is set for season 2's interspecies struggle for survival, going beyond cultural competition between human factions. Such an ending does not affirm the reproductive cyborg and suggests that the pursuit of heterocoital reproduction by the wrong bodies leads to its hijacking by monsters.

Even though the end results differ, in *Raised by Wolves,* as in *Blade Runner 2049,* resolutions to the fears about failures of heterocoital reproductive order indicate that nontraditional reproduction may specifically threaten the ideas and values of patriarchy. In both, we see the importance of known paternity, as the biological father determines the child's identity and belonging. In *Raised by Wolves,* such a father is the source of a child's nonnegotiable otherness, and in *Blade Runner 2049,* Deckard legitimizes a hybrid child as human. *Blade Runner 2049,* for example, constructs Deckard's right to appropriate the child as "natural" through heterocoital discourse, by the power of his heterocoitus with Rachel, which trumps the right of the Tyrell and Wallace corporations to Rachel as a patented technology, or the right of replicants—her kind, race, or species—to their genealogy in her child. Deckard shapes and appropriates the futurity genetically encoded in his biological child. At the same time, the alien nature of Mother's child in *Raised by Wolves* is established by the eels' belonging to the father-serpent, through a discovery of the outcome of the deceptive heterocoital act. This discovery changes the meaning of the impostor's claim that Mother carries the future of humanity inside her. When she understands that human futurity is hijacked by the planet's original form of life and human continuity is in peril, she, as Lt. Joshi is in *Blade Runner,* has no compassion for the child and is ready to kill it to save humans. In both films, known paternity determines the identity and belonging of the child that defines the futurity of the human world. In his interview, Guzikowski shared that the idea for *Raised by Wolves* was prompted by how closely his own children were integrated with technology and that the starting point for the show was the perspective of Campion, a lonely child on an alien planet with his human siblings dead and his parents obviously nonhuman (Guzikowski 2020b). "It's just starting from that perspective, that kind of empty, 'What now?'" says Guzikowski, who immediately follows with "But throughout it all, we're going to see it through the lens of this family" (Guzikowski 2020b). In a different interview, he stated that the intended main themes of the show were "the importance of family . . . whatever shape or form it may take" and "faith . . . be it faith in technology or faith in religion and the search for purpose and meaning" (Guzikowski 2020a). When crafting the aesthetic of the show, he was looking for "the feeling [of] . . . old Grimm's Fairy Tales and the Old Testament stories or Greek myths," which activate "some genetic trigger we have built inside of us" (Guzikowski 2020b). This quote shows the interconnectedness of nature, technology, religion, and culture in the show's author's imagination, and even though he acknowledges "whatever forms" family and faith can have, he says in the same breath, "Whether it's the nuclear family or us as a species, in essence that's what we are" (Guzikowski 2020a). The nuclear family and species continuity are equalized and connected by a *genetic* tie to the narratives we tell about them. This is the biocultural imagination at work.

If we imagine culture as transmitted in its totality through biological reproduction and as reliant on uninterrupted genealogies, potential revisions to either the biological or cultural meanings of reproduction may stir the fear of human extinction and the desire to destroy the Other who threatens humans. In *A.I. Artificial Intelligence,* this desire is encapsulated in the phenomenon of the Flesh Fair—a public spectacle of robot demolition. To justify David's destruction, the announcer says that robot children like David were created to "steal your hearts, to replace your children"—and thus inflects nontraditional kinship both with an anxiety over culturally suspect, deceptive affect and with the sense of an ending for the human species. The film's world of the future confirms these fears as it portrays the world populated by mechas—likely a consequence of the technological revision to human reproductive and affective practices ushered in by David and his replicas. In the context of the film, such a revision results in the disappearance of humans—an expression of technophobia rooted in the understanding of technology as the humans' Other, which is a way of thinking that does not allow for imagining nontraditional kinship formations as fully human and culturally acceptable in their own right, only as imitations of biological kinship. What would it take to think about origins and kinship, technology and biology, biology and culture differently? Where could it take us?

CONCLUSION

One is too few, but two are too many.
One is too few, and two is only one possibility.
—Donna Haraway, "A Cyborg Manifesto" (55, 56)

Several years ago, this book started as a way to examine reasons for the double binds of adoption widely represented in the cultural production and scholarship around the subject: among them, the need for the adoptees to negotiate the degrees of their belonging with the biological and adoptive families; the cultural demand that the adoptive family both imitates and differentiates itself from the heterocoital nuclear one; the pressure to simultaneously let go and be a parent, experienced by the heterocoital parents of adoptees; to name a few. The analysis of assisted-reproduction films in this book shows that similar constraints, albeit not the same ones, have emerged in cultural discourses around other forms of nontraditional reproduction. The ideas that this book has developed suggest that double binds generated by the demand to imitate "real" kinship originate in the commitment of Western cultures to the symbolic order grounded in heterocoital reproduction. The primacy of heterocoital reproduction in its patriarchal iteration is maintained by patriarchal institutions, even as the ways in which humans reproduce themselves change. This book's analysis of representations of adoption and ARTs shows that anyone who wants to be recognized as a human subject and a person would still be compelled to anchor their selfhood in a heterocoital origin and a congruity between such origin and the family in which one is raised. When such congruity splinters, heterocoital patriarchal cultures insist on understanding and naming new ways of reproduction through old, heterocoital kinship tropes. This is when the double binds emerge.

Double binds indicate that traditional kinship practices and cultural scripts for selfhood and human interrelatedness based on them retain the power to structure the lives of people who have been brought to life and raised in nontraditional kinship arrangements. This book's analysis of adoption and ART representations shows that heterocoital reproduction has produced an ideology, a set of ideas, that shapes our thinking about origin, identity, belonging, kinship, and larger social institutions and processes. And it also shows that our imaginations are challenged by changes in the reproductive landscape. Heterosexuality and the nuclear family form can no longer comfortably accommodate all ways of nontraditional reproduction. Same-sex families can now reproduce biologically through gamete donation and surrogacy. In-vitro gametogenesis (IVG) can create gametes out of any adult cell, which means that same-sex couples can have a child that is biogenetically related to both partners; a single person can use their own material to create a child through a process that is not cloning; or even a group of people can produce children that will be their genetic progeny. Anchoring human identity and belonging in biogenetic origin understood as equivalent to "the natural ways of doing things" is becoming more and more complicated. Currently, staying faithful to the heterocoital reproduction metaphor still "allows new technology to coevolve with existing sexual, gender, and kinship norms, adding a degree of flexibility to the reproduction of reproduction, while largely keeping the structure of bilateral, biological kinship norms intact" (Franklin 6–7). In other words, the heterocoital order still seems resilient, and families that more explicitly challenge heterocoital reproduction and heterosexuality can be pulled into the work of kinship normalization that brings the identities of the families and children in line with heterocoital cultural scripts. But, as much work within critical adoption studies (CAS) has demonstrated, when heterocoital origins and families are imitated in nontraditional reproduction situations, it may produce private suffering and precarity around one's social status.

Given the growing frequency of assisted reproduction, the cultural significance of biological (read: heterocoital) origins—well known to scholars in CAS—begins to matter more and more to larger categories of people. IVF and other assisted reproductive technologies are the precursors of the world in which heterocoital origins, even in the case of a fusion of male and female gametes in a petri dish, may not be universally available or valuable for all humans. Come to think of it, ARTs that aim to mimic heterocoital reproduction in pursuit of biological and genetic relatedness or its imitation at the level of conception, take us further away from normative ways of kinship relatedness than adoption does. While adoption can still be parsed in terms of biologically related and social parents, and in the case of adoption, a child still has two heterocoital genitors and thus a heterocoital origin, ARTs may further amplify genealogical uncertainty around the biological component of reproduction. Some ARTs fudge the point of conception to the degree that the biological mechanism of such reproduction cannot be narratively converted into the conventional heterocoital origin considered universal for humans. While it is still possible to "naturalize" IVF, for example, by narrating it in terms of heterocoital reproduction, such technologies as induced pluripotent stem cells[1] may more obviously establish reproductive difference as a fact of life. From CAS's vantage point, we should be alert to the problems such difference may create for many if we continue to make sense of nontraditional forms of being and kinship "through [old] ideas" (Strathern 4) that assume heterocoital reproduction to be a universal and necessary condition for human personhood.

But if the primacy of heterocoital origin is decentered, we could better discern the importance of the heterocoital logic to the patriarchy. Chapter 3 touched upon the role of the concept of known paternity for family formations based on heterocoital origin. The idea that known paternity is the basis of patriarchal institutions was developed by Mary O'Brien, who also outlined the importance of analyzing reproduction as a social process instead of relegating it to the realm of "dumb" nature. Instead of looking at reproduction as a natural, and hence immutable, phenomenon, we could subject it to scrutiny as always vested in social and cultural framing provided by the patriarchy. O'Brien, for example, observes that while other "natural functions" like "eating, sexuality, and dying" have received a lot of attention in what she calls "male-stream thought," birth, as a phenomenon, has been neglected by major philosophers (1981, 20–21). Even analysis that aims to critique patriarchal perspectives on reproduction and kinship may retain their commitment to the patriarchy-inflected conceptual apparatus. Sara Dorow and Amy Swiffen's review of new kinship studies' critiques of "heteronormative assumptions that underpin anthropological concepts of kinship" (564) shows that "new kinship studies' theorizations of heteronormativity" may still "reproduce[e] [it] 'even' amidst hybrid, multiple family forms" (564). As an example of a critique of such tendencies, they use the work of Evelyn Blackwood, who has demonstrated that "the absent presence of the 'patriarchal man' [still] structures

1. Induced pluripotent stem cells are skin or blood cells reprogrammed back to their stem-cell state, so they become capable of growing into any kind of cell, including egg and sperm precursors.

concepts intended to capture alternative kinship arrangements," as it does in the idea of "matrifocal," understood as defined against the "organizing term" of the patriarchy (565).

Moving away from the tenet that heterocoital origin is a universal human condition paves the way to more complexity in analyses of reproduction. It may create additional texture in understanding adoption and its comparisons to ARTs. For example, while it seems logical to look at ARTs through ideas developed around another form of nontraditional family created through adoption, and, indeed, there exists a certain continuity, the analogy is far from direct. In conversations about assisted reproduction, analogies with adoption are typically brought up when they touch upon the origins of an ART-conceived person and the consequences of not knowing or being confused about them.[2] Diane Ehrensaft, for instance, is urging psychologist-practitioners who help people that undergo conception using ARTs to look toward adoption as a field where a lot of work in negotiating identity, belonging, and origins has already been done. She points to the long-term effects of disclosure of the child's "roots" (2014, 35) and urges these professionals to reconsider secrecy around the information about participants in a child's conception and birth, to avoid identity confusion issues. At the same time, Kimberly Leighton, a critical adoption studies scholar, suggests that "adoptees and people who were donor-conceived [may not] necessarily suffer—*if* they suffer at all—from the same phenomena" (2014, 257). She argues that in the case of anonymous gamete donation (AGD), such analogizing "based on the harms of secrecy and the harm of genealogical bewilderment" (242) leads to "geneteciz[ing of] the adoptees' experiences" and obscures the specificity of their adopted condition (242). If we look at adoption and AGD as different reproductive processes (which they are if we consider heterocoital origin as the basis of comparison), we can see, as Leighton suggests, that the adoptee's need to know may be driven by the need to understand, for example, the reasons for relinquishment, including the possible lack of birth mother's love, which in AGD case may not be in question. Comparing adoptees and ART-conceived people, then, produces "an erasure from the experience of adoption of the difference that being adopted makes . . . [and] a foreclosure on how being adopted might engender alternative ways of understanding the meaning of relatedness" (261). By the same token, the experience of an ART-conceived individual may be eclipsed by the analogy that relies on heterocoital discourse even as it aims to compare ways of reproduction that destabilize it.

---

2. On comparisons of the effects of adoption and ART conception, also see Witt; Blake et al.

At the same time, adoption studies' knowledge can surely help an understanding of the logic of ARTs' co-optation within the existing heterocoital scripts. The social imperative for the adoptive family to be "just like" the biological family serves to reimagine adoption in terms of heterocoital reproduction, and it demands that the adoptee confirm their heterocoital origin by knowing that they have heterocoital (a.k.a. birth) parents. In adoption, the transfer of the child to the adoptive parents is understood as a shift in social parenting, while the adoptee's biological origin remains the same as a non-adopted individual's. In this way, the culturally required "need to know" one's birth parents serves to reinforce the primacy of heterocoital reproduction even in nontraditional family-making. The analogy between ARTs and adoption piggybacks on this conceptual move and reinvents it further as it likens ART conception to an already established idea of the heterocoital "normalcy" of adoption, even though the logic of the normalization process has differences. While some forms of ART conception can be easily folded back into the heterocoital logic (e.g., when the sperm of the social father, not donor, is used for an IUI), others (e.g., AGD or surrogacy) require further conceptual work to align themselves with heterocoital imperatives. For instance, an equivalency between adoptees' and ART-conceived individuals' rights to know their origins may parentize donors, so to speak, and imagine them as birth parents, but it may be an unwelcome development for many donors. The complexities and differences between modes of reproduction, most of which splinter biocultural consistency of kinship, parenting, and individual origin, tend to be subsumed within the heterocoital imaginary, where all "irregularities" of reproductive process are refashioned in terms of heterocoital, nuclear family. But the consequences of ARTs for cultural ideas about identity and belonging cannot be imagined as simply an extension of adoption-related ideas.

To reiterate, adoption reinvents traditional kinship, but it still keeps it rooted in heterocoital reproduction. In other words, the heterocoital basis of biological identity remains constant, and adoption does not challenge heterocoital origin as *the* anchor of human identity. But many forms of ARTs do, and they introduce more participants into the reproductive process than the two heterocoital genitors. At the same time, ART families may often, though not always, "pass" more easily for heterocoital than adoptive families do, and thus more easily "naturalize" nontraditional kinship built on technologically assisted reproduction. The outcome of such naturalization often silences and de-recognizes reproductive participants. ARTs also produce anxieties over the child's belonging, given the increased involvement of third parties in the process that used to be owned by two biological genitors. Families who work with donors may resist kinning by renaming them in a language that medicalizes them and minimizes their potential to be construed as kin (e.g., *donor, surrogate*). Writing about the psychoanalytical effects of ARTs, Ehrensaft (2014) observes that the oedipal triangle expands to a circle and families need to contend with a different paradigm of oedipal development. While she points out that in a culture that privileges genetic family ties, the titles of mother and father need to be applied to people who "who intended to have a baby" (36) in order to stabilize the oedipal triangle, she also predicts that both parents and the child may deal with other individuals involved in reproduction in ways that may restructure oedipal patterns of affect and belonging. ART reproduction may raise questions about the ownership of a child or of biomaterial, the place of the third parties in the family structure, or the custody of abandoned frozen embryos. These are new, emerging issues that may exceed the frame of heterocoital narratives used to constitute identities and families. As taken-for-granted family ties become insufficient to account for one's place in the world and the network of human relationships, attention may gravitate toward the concept of belonging, rather than kinship. Ehrensaft, for example, warns that failure to account for changes in kinship configurations caused by ARTs may "not only render ourselves out of synch with changing realities; we may create harm by inferring, interpreting, or imposing pathology or loss when there may be none" (2014, 22). Expanding the vocabulary of belonging, beyond heterocoital kinship, could help us imagine nontraditional reproduction and family, not in terms of "heterocoital lack" but on their own terms.

For example, as ways of transcending the primacy of the heterocoital narrative, CAS scholars have already begun deconstructions of "family," or consolidations of new subjectivities of nontraditional family's members, such as the adoptee's. Sayres Rudy thinks that biocentrism as well as its critique in adoption studies position the adoptee as a "biodivergent minorit[y]" (209) that is imagined in terms of lack in both discourses and is thus deconstituted as a subject and object of inquiry. Even discourses aimed at reinstating the adoptee's experience seem to obscure it by imagining it as a deprivation of what people raised by their heterocoital genitors have. Rudy also theorizes persistent ambivalence of both genetic and affective-social kinship, pointing out that "the 'blood' metaphor" has been a "symbolic abstraction that gave affective significance to nonbiological social attachments" and that such transfer was possible because "traditional kinship was never literally, only metaphorically, genetic and consanguineous" (216). Such dematerialization of blood represents "supra-genetic communal desire" (216) and "blood and love metaphors serve the identical purpose: repressing the plurality of actually-existing kinship relations in order to stabilize distinct articulations of biocentric social order" (215). In order to subvert such thinking, Leighton argues, and "to promote choices of how to organize one's family . . . we need to challenge directly the claim that one is necessarily harmed by one's genetic ignorance" (2013, 55). To complicate the conversation about the harms of adoption, Emily Hipchen offers an invitation to recognize that "no one suffers from adoption as *a specific category of experience,* [even though] many people might actually suffer in their adoptive families" (2023). She invites adoption scholars to analyze what she names "the feeling of adoption" as a "feeling of difference" to understand more thoroughly why adoption is seen as traumatic (2023).

An acceptance of the impossibility to wrap all nontraditional reproduction into the heterocoital model invites deeper scrutiny of potential reproductive futurities and consequences of forms of adoption and ARTs for human life. For example, current feminist thought considers the possibility of crystallized patriarchy as an outcome of ARTs' development (chapter 4 engaged with this idea), but feminist thinkers are divided about the significance of non-heterocoital reproduction for women. In *New Reproductive Technologies,* Carla Lam classifies feminist response to ARTs into three approaches: the "embracers" (41), who celebrate technology as liberation from the oppressive reproduction process; the "resistors" (41), who question the seemingly liberatory potential of assisted reproduction for women by claiming that it alienates women from their embodied experience and gives men an opportunity to denaturalize nature-woman in order to gain reproductive power to which they have had more limited access; and the "equivocals" (65), who aim to negotiate a middle-ground stance that takes into account specific intersectionalities of women in understanding the value and threat of ARTs. As an "equivocal," Dana S. Belu, for example, says that IVF may empower individual women, but not all of them as a class (26). ARTs challenge heterocoital paradigm by separating coitus from reproduction at the risk of alienating women from the childbearing and labor process. This may result in *disembodiment* of women due to their alienation from the reproductive process, and, following suit of fetus-imaging technologies, women may be reimagined as vessels, donors, and replaceable body parts. ARTs may become a way to treat male infertility, and women's bodies will be invaded and taxed to alleviate problems experienced by men and children, as Irma van der Ploeg argues in *Prosthetic Bodies.* Technopatriarchy can reinvent human reproduction along the lines of its cultural dogmas.

But there is also a promise that arises from the reproductive estrangement that women may experience in the absence of gestation and labor as necessary stages in reproduction. While it might break the natural link to species continuity that O'Brien theorizes as a central quality of female reproductive consciousness, the very break may make it explicit that such link has been taken for granted and the consequences of its potential dissolution remained largely unexamined. Continuation of life as a model for human temporality based on women's reproductive consciousness has always been present in culture as an alternative to patriarchy. Now it has a chance to become more explicit and foundational. In the new reproductive landscape, male reproductive consciousness may not change qualitatively (unless a man becomes capable of gestation and birth), only in the degree of control over the means of reproduction. Women, however, will have a choice of reproductive experience that is likely to change their reproductive consciousness. To avoid universalization of male reproductive consciousness, O'Brien suggests that women engage in more deliberate cultural mediation of their now multifaceted relationship to nature, but in a way different from men's alienation. Given that the patriarchy is not interested in giving "any historical meaning to the need to create social relations of reproduction, muttering darkly about biological determinism and reductionism" (16)—a legacy of the "ages of totally involuntary pregnancy" (16), O'Brien believed feminists can develop their own culture in order to meet the new "material change in that combination of consciousness and experience which is the process of reproduction" (160–61). She pointed out that the heterocoital ideology of patriarchy is not going to concern itself with the development of a new kinship lexicon, since it does not "recogniz[e] the family as a historical phenomenon," thinking of it instead as a product of "modes of production" or "free personal choice" (17). So it falls to the women's "second nature" to establish "the value of life as such" (O'Brien 1989, 15) as the basis of "a different political understanding and relation to the natural and social realms" ushered by the new reproductive technologies (Brodribb 260). Proponents of such thinking believe that it is possible to see ARTs as an opportunity to reinvent the way we are reproducing the world both biologically and culturally and create a new set of social relationships around reproduction that do not reinscribe the ideology of the "universal man." For instance, in her reflection on possibilities for feminist futurity and continuity, Sommer Brodribb looks toward O'Brien and Irigaray, whose feminist sensibilities might help invent a "different relationship to death and to the 'other'" than those spawned by "Heidegger's Being-Unto-Death" (258, 257). Brodribb writes that Irigaray and O'Brien, each in their own but interlocking ways, develop philosophies that "generate a feminist future and presence" (258), a future "which is not measured by the transcendence of death but by the call to birth of the self and the other" (Irigaray, qtd. in Brodribb 258).

Such thinking overlaps with the goals of critical posthumanism in its revision of narcissistic anthropocentrism and hierarchy-producing dualities. In a conversation about reproduction, posthumanism's focus on the relationship between humans and technology becomes relevant as a methodology that could help transcend the double binds of nontraditional reproduction, the danger of reproductive difference between "real" and "artificial" origins, and the idea that heterocoital kinship is the only ("real") one. Critical (also called "philosophical")[3] posthumanism revises the relationship between humans and technology and encourages a movement beyond the idea that technology is "the other" of humanity and a tool that humans wield to change the natural conditions of their environment. Instead, it offers the idea of technogenesis[4]—an acceptance of human "nature" as co-emergent with techniques humans use. Bruno Latour's articulation of this idea abandons understanding of technology as "socially constructed," in other words, as created to carry social relationships and inscribed with social meanings (793). He suggests that human-technology relationship is a constant "swap[ping of] properties" between humans and nonhumans in the process of "socialization of nonhumans" (791, 793). In other words, technologies and humans act together and upon each other as co-creators of each other in each iteration of what is commonly understood as progress or development. In terms of reproduction, this idea tells us that we cannot divide it into categories of natural and nontraditional any more than we can posit heterocoital origin as an unquestionably universal and stable basis of humanity. While ARTs are seen as obviously technological, the perspective of technogenesis allows for seeing all human reproduction, including adoption, as such. Given that human conception and birth have always been mediated with techniques and by Latour's "socialized nonhumans," whether through conception or birthing rituals or the use of the forceps or drugs during delivery, can we really think of human reproduction as natural, even if it is heterocoital? If we see reproduction as a mediated process, it may well be that heterocoital origin and kinship are not the only possibility. This opens space for considering ways of reproduction outside of the dualistic (traditional/nontraditional) framework that is designed to produce reproductive hierarchies.

Such an approach is bound to produce anxieties in cultures that have relied on the Enlightenment-based humanism-inflected thinking to assert the value of human life. So far, *humanity*, as a category of identity, has served well as the foundational concept for extending human rights and battling oppression. Rosi Braidotti points out, however, that the very fact that "not all of us can say . . . that we have always been human" (2013, 1) reveals the instability

3. See Ferrando (2019) for distinctions between different schools of thought that have used the term "posthuman."

4. Katherine Hayles unpacks the term in her book *How We Think* (2012).

of the human-nonhuman duality as a foundation for equality, because the definition of "the human" is a matter of social consensus, and, historically, it has been reserved for whomever was recognized as human at that time. Within the humanist framework, *humanity* has signaled which lives are worth life and nurture and which ones become forms of living death. *Humanity* is deconstructed by critical posthumanism through a critique of exclusionary dualism that differentiates between humans and nonhumans. The difference of this approach from dehumanization and anti-humanism is its affirmation of the value of all life, which undermines the idea of hierarchical difference and allows for directing attention and recognition to previously neglected phenomena. Francesca Ferrando describes the revisions to the humanist framework offered by critical posthumanism as "post exclusivism: an empirical philosophy of mediation which offers a reconciliation of existence in its broadest significations" and revises the ways of thinking that have historically produced inequalities and social hierarchies (29). In that, critical posthumanism aligns with Donna Haraway's concept of cyborgism that rejects the idea of definable origin (2007, 56), and of the "Chthulucene" that "entangles myriad temporalities and spatialities and myriad intra-active entities-in-assemblages—including the more-than-human, other-than-human, inhuman, and human-as-humus" (2016, 101). The blurring of the boundaries between artificial/natural, human/nonhuman, alive/nonliving becomes a way to curb the construction of difference as a means of oppression.

Together with race, gender, ability, and other more familiar markers of humanity, reproductive difference (which intersects with other categories) requires increased attention in the era of biotechnological advancements. When women are not guaranteed the "natural" connection to the child and future and children are not guaranteed a "natural" anchor to identity and belonging, when biology becomes a discourse subject to editing, the category of the human that has historically been used to determine the biopolitical value of individual lives will need redefinition or at least a culturally shared understanding of its fluidity and dependence on social consensus about the meaning of humanity and the value of certain lives. We can begin to deliberately revise the ways we think of identity, kinship, and belonging, based on an understanding of technology not as a tool but as a constitutive part of human genesis. The emerging reproductive consciousness, then, may acknowledge that assisted reproduction is a concern not only for those who participate in it but for our shared human condition at the age of assisted reproduction. Adoption may change as an institution focused on reaffirming the primacy of heterocoital kinship and may no longer be haunted by cultural scripts that continue to see it as the "second-best" or, with the availability of ARTs, "third-best" option. The adoptee would be culturally perceived no longer as a substitute for a potential biological child but, rather, an integral part of a family that can only exist as an adoptive one; there is no other possibility that could haunt the adoptive family as an unrealized potential. ARTs may not be seen as an instrument of achieving the heterocoital family persistently considered natural and the only one. Instead, it will be seen as a means to achieve the experience of reproduction understood and explored in multiple, uniquely experienced ways. Adopted and ART-reproduced humans will be free to stop constantly negotiating their status or passing for heterocoitally reproduced and instead focus on exploring their own condition of reproduction, which cultures would see as "one of many" and not "the other." Some of this thinking is already present in, for example, the idea that adoptive transracial and transnational families are hybridized by the act of adoption. Instead of perceiving itself as a family that harbors "the other," the whole family is transracially or transnationally adoptive. Such perspective can free us to pay attention to the qualities and qualia of each coming-into-being, rather than erasing, suppressing, and reinterpreting them toward the demands of the heterocoital framework.

Understandably, such perspective may produce deep anxieties about existential threats to humanity because it challenges established ideas about human nature and human subjecthood. As Donna Haraway explains, hierarchical dualistic thought locks the subject, "the One," who identifies themselves in terms of their difference from "the other," in "a dialectic of apocalypse with the [dominated and erased] other" (2007, 55). In this dyad, the other remains reduced and invisible even to the One, the liberal autonomous subject of the humanist paradigm. This happens because the visibility of the other is always a threat to "the [imagined] autonomy of the self"—the main tenet of Western human subjecthood (55). The existence of the other needs to be constantly derealized because even though the other is required for the One to come into being via the dialectic of difference, the recognition of the other means the end of the raison d'être of the One. Dualistic thought, for example, maintains the paradigm in which the heterocoital family is locked in "the dialectic of apocalypse" with its others—adoption and ART reproduction—whose emancipation is only imagined as successful imitation. Such apocalyptical thinking could manifest in, for instance, understanding the central idea of this book as advocating an abolition of the heterocoital family, while, in fact, the book is calling for expanding the register of recognized kinds of origins and kinships that are valuable in themselves, not as imitations of the heterocoital kinship. In other words, "one is too few" (Haraway 2007, 55). The broadening of the dualistic perspective does not have to end in relativism or postmodernist celebration of differences without an end. Instead, we need to cultivate deep attention to the meaning of reproduction in the changing technological landscape without dualistic blinders. Perhaps we can begin imagining nontraditional reproductive practices as culturally viable if we begin to see technology as an always present condition of human becoming and think of biology not as an immutable natural "law" but as a historicized "complex web of [knowledge-producing] practices" that we can "participate in and make better" (Haraway 1996, 323). If we reconceptualize technology and the human as enmeshed and mutually constitutive, nontraditional reproduction and kinship may have the power to revise and enrich the heterocoital symbolic order, our selfhoods, and the way we relate to each other and the world.

ACKNOWLEDGMENTS

This book would have been impossible without the steady support of my critical adoption studies colleagues and the publishing team at The Ohio State University Press.

I would like to extend my gratitude to Emily Hipchen for many a stimulating discussion of ideas about adoption and ART and for the help with naming this book. Our conversations and her feedback have given this project the energy to move forward. I am also extremely grateful to Margaret Homans for her belief in the importance of these ideas and her insightful feedback. My peer review readers have offered thoughtful feedback, and I am grateful for their input, which has made this book better.

I would like to thank all of my critical adoption studies colleagues for shaping the field of study that has become our intellectual home. Our conversations during conferences and individual exchanges have created the space where scholarship like this matters.

Support from OSUP's Kristen Elias Rowley, especially through the COVID years, has been invaluable and unwavering. Thank you.

My deepest thanks to my friends and family for supporting me at every turn, especially to my husband, Alex, for understanding and sharing the ups and downs of the writer's process.

Special thanks to the University Committee on Research in the Humanities and Social Sciences (UCRHSS) at Princeton for funding that supported the late stages of this manuscript's development.

Portions of this book first appeared in earlier forms as "The Power to 'Make Live': Biopolitics and Reproduction in *Blade Runner 2049*," *Adoption and Culture*, vol. 7, no. 2, 2019, pp. 169–75; "Slouching towards Old-Fashioned: How the Heterocoital Family Shapes the Future of Reproduction," a review of Kathryn Jenkins's *Private Life*, *Adoption and Culture*, vol. 7, no. 1, 2019, pp. 141–51; "Adoption in Steven Spielberg's *A.I.*: Kinship in Posthuman Context," *Adoption and Culture*, vol. 6, no. 1, 2018, pp. 182–205; and "*Orphan* and *A Member of the Family*: Disability and Secrecy in Narratives of Disrupted Eastern European Adoption," *Adoption and Culture*, vol. 3, 2012, pp. 7–32.

WORKS CITED

Ahmed, Sara. 2014. *The Cultural Politics of Emotion.* Edinburgh UP.

A.I. Artificial Intelligence. 2001. Directed by Steven Spielberg, Warner Bros.

Altman, Rick. 1999. *Film/Genre.* British Film Institute.

Anagnost, Ann. 2000. "Scenes of Misrecognition: Maternal Citizenship in the Age of Transnational Adoption." *Positions: East Asia Cultures Critique,* vol. 8, no. 2, pp. 389–421.

Atterton, Peter. 2015. *"More Human than Human": "Blade Runner" and Being-Toward-Death.* Routledge.

The Bad Seed. 1956. Directed by Mervyn LeRoy, Warner Bros.

Barnes, Colin, and Geoffrey Mercer. 2003. *Disability.* Polity.

Bawarshi, Anis. 2000. "The Genre Function." *College English,* vol. 62, no. 3, pp. 335–60.

Blade Runner. 1982. Directed by Ridley Scott, Warner Bros.

Blade Runner. 1992. Directed by Ridley Scott, director's cut, Warner Bros.

Blade Runner 2049. 2017. Directed by Denis Villeneuve, Warner Bros.

Blake, Lucy, et al. 2014. "The Families of Assisted Reproduction and Adoption." *Family-Making: Contemporary Ethical Challenges,* edited by Francoise Baylis and Carolyn McLeod, Oxford UP, pp. 64–88.

Belu, Dana S. 2017. *Heidegger, Reproductive Technology, and the Motherless Age.* Palgrave McMillan.

Berebitsky, Julie. 2004. "Redefining 'Real' Motherhood: Representations of Adoptive Mothers, 1900–1950." *Imagining Adoption: Essays on Literature and Culture,* edited by Marianne Novy, U of Michigan P, pp. 83–96.

Blackwood, Evelyn. 2008. "The Specter of the Patriarchal Man." *American Ethnologist,* vol. 32, no. 1, pp. 42–45.

Bordo, Susan. 2002. "All of Us Are Real: Old Images in a New World of Adoption." *The Adoption Issue,* special issue of *Tulsa Studies in Women's Literature,* vol. 21, no. 2, pp. 319–31.

Bradshaw, Peter. 2012. "*Mother and Child* Review." *The Guardian,* 5 Jan., https://www.theguardian.com/film/2012/jan/05/mother-and-child-film-review.

Braidotti, Rosi. 2006. "Posthuman, All Too Human: Towards a New Process Ontology." *Theory, Culture, and Society,* vol. 23, nos. 7–8, pp. 197–208.

Braidotti, Rosi. 2013. *The Posthuman.* Polity.

Briggs, Laura. 2017. *How All Politics Became Reproductive Politics: From Welfare Reform to Foreclosure to Trump.* U of California P.

Brodribb, Somer. 1992. "The Birth of Time: Generation(s) and Genealogy in Mary O'Brien and Luce Irigaray." *Time and Society,* vol. 1, no. 2, pp. 257–70.

Brooks, Peter. 1995. *The Melodramatic Imagination.* Yale UP.

Burke, Rennie, et al. 2021. "How Do Individuals Who Were Conceived Through the Use of Donor Technologies Feel About the Nature of Their Conception?" *Biotechnology,* 1 Apr., *Harvard Medical School,* https://bioethics.hms.harvard.edu/journal/donor-technology.

Burfoot, Annette. 2014. "Revisiting Mary O'Brien: Reproductive Consciousness and Liquid Maternity." *Socialist Studies,* vol. 10, no. 1, pp. 174–90.

Bussing, Sabine. 1987. *Aliens in the Home: The Child in Horror Fiction.* Greenwood Press.

Butler, Judith. 2004. *Undoing Gender.* Routledge.

Callahan, Cynthia. 2011. *Kin of Another Kind: Transracial Adoption in American Literature.* U of Michigan P.

Carangelo, Lori. 2015. *The Adoption and Donor Conception Factbook: The Only Comprehensive Source of U.S. and Global Data on the Invisible Families of Adoption, Foster Care and Donor Conception.* Genealogical Publishing Company / Clearfield Company.

Carp, Wayne. 2002a. "Adoption, Blood Kinship, Stigma, and the Adoption Reform Movement: A Historical Perspective." *Law and Society Review,* vol. 36, no. 2, pp. 433–60.

Carp, Wayne. 2002b. "A Historical Overview of American Adoption." *Adoption in America: Historical Perspectives,* edited by Wayne Carp, Michigan UP, pp. 1–26.

Carroll, Noel. 1990. *The Philosophy of Horror; or, Paradoxes of the Heart.* Routledge.

Cartwright, Lisa. 2003. "Photographs of 'Waiting Children': The Transnational Adoption Market." *Social Text,* vol. 21 no. 1, pp. 83–109. https://muse.jhu.edu/article/41634.

Catfish in Black Bean Sauce. 2000. Directed by Chi Muoi Lo, Black Hawk Entertainment.

Chambers, Deborah. 2006. *New Social Ties: Contemporary Connections in a Fragmented Society.* Springer.

Chassagnol, Monique. "Masks and Masculinity in James Barrie's *Peter Pan.*" *Ways of Being Male: Representing Masculinities in Children's Literature,* edited by John Stephens. pp. 200–215.

Clarke, Cath. 2018. "*Private Life* Review—Netflix Fertility Comedy Is Painfully Funny." 5 Oct., https://www.theguardian.com/film/2018/oct/05/private-life-review-netflix-fertility-comedy-paul-giamatti.

"Dave Thomas Foundation for Adoption Poll: January 2002." 2002. Conducted by Harris Initiative. *Roper,* https://doi.org/10.25940/ROPER-31109089.

Deleyto, Celestino. 2013. "Humor and Erotic Utopia: The Intimate Scenarios of Romantic Comedy." *A Companion to Film Comedy,* edited by Andrew Horton and Johanna E. Rapf, Wiley Blackwell, pp. 175–95.

Delivery Man. 2013. Directed by Ken Scott. Walt Disney Studios Motion Pictures.

"*Delivery Man.*" Film synopsis. *IMDB,* https://www.imdb.com/title/tt2387559/.

"*Delivery Man.*" Film synopsis. *Rotten Tomatoes,* https://www.rottentomatoes.com/m/delivery_man.

"*The Delivery Man.*" Product description. *Amazon,* https://www.amazon.com/Delivery-Man-Vince-Vaughn/dp/B00I8R4DNC.

Dolan, Jill. 2010. Review of *The Kids Are Alright. The Feminist Spectator,* 30 July, https://feministspectator.princeton.edu/2010/07/30/the-kids-are-all-right/.

Dorow, Sara K. 2006. *Transnational Adoption: A Cultural Economy of Race, Gender, and Kinship.* New York UP.

Dorow, Sara K., and Amy Swiffen. 2009. "Blood and Desire: The Secret of Heteronormativity in Adoption Narratives of Culture." *American Ethnologist,* vol. 36, no. 3, pp. 563–73.

Du Bois, W. E. B. 1903. "The Talented Tenth." In *The Negro Problem,* James Pott and Company, pp. 31–77.

Duggan, Lisa. 2002. "The New Homonormativity: The Sexual Politics of Neoliberalism." *Materializing Democracy: Toward a Revitalized Cultural Policy,* edited by Russ Canstronovo and Dana D. Nelson, Duke University Press, pp. 175–94.

Eaklor, Vicki. 2008. *Queer America: A GLBT History of the 20th Century.* Greenwood Press.

Ebert, Roger. 1995. Review of *Losing Isaiah. Roger Ebert,* 17 Mar., https://www.rogerebert.com/reviews/losing-isaiah-1995.

Ebert, Roger. 2005. "*Syriana* Pours Oil on Troubled Sands." *Roger Ebert,* 8 Dec. https://www.rogerebert.com/reviews/syriana-2005.

Ebert, Roger. 2010. "But the Moms Have Some Issues." *Roger Ebert,* 7 July, https://www.rogerebert.com/reviews/the-kids-are-all-right-2010.

Edelstein, David. 2018. "Kathryn Hahn Is Dazzling in *Private Life,* a Tale About Makeshift Families." *Vulture,* 20 Jan., https://www.vulture.com/2018/01/review-private-life-is-a-dazzling-comedy-about-families.html.

Ehrensaft, Diane. 2014. "Family Complexes and Oedipal Circles: Mothers, Fathers, Babies, Donors, and Surrogates." *Psychoanalytic Aspects of Assisted Reproductive Technology,* edited by Mali Mann, Taylor & Francis Group, pp. 19–44.

Embryo. 1976. Directed by Ralph Nelson, Sandy Howard Productions and Plura Service Company.

"Evan B. Donaldson Adoption Institute Poll: July 1997." 1997. Conducted by Princeton Survey Research Associates. *Roper,* https://doi.org/10.25940/ROPER-31107064.

Everett, Wendy. 2005. "Fractal Films and the Architecture of Complexity." *Studies in European Cinema,* vol. 2, no. 3, pp. 159–71.

Fahy, Thomas. 2012. *The Philosophy of Horror.* UP of Kentucky.

Fakin' da Funk. 1997. Directed by Tim Chey, Octillion Entertainment.

False Positive. 2021. Directed by John Lee, A24.

Fanon, Frantz. 1963. "Concerning Violence." *The Wretched of the Earth,* by Fanon. Translated by Constance Farrington, Grove Press, pp. 35–94.

Fedosik, Marina. 2009a. "Genealogical Ambiguity and Racial Identity: Adoption and Passing in Kate Chopin's 'Desiree's Baby' and Jessie Redmon Fauset's 'The Sleeper Wakes.'" *America and the Black Body: Identity Politics in Print and Visual Culture,* edited by Carol Henderson, Fairleigh Dickinson UP, pp. 180–98.

Fedosik, Marina. 2009b. *Representations of Transnational Adoption in Contemporary Literature and Film.* University of Delaware, PhD dissertation.

Ferrando, Fracesca. 2013. "Posthumanism, Transhumanism, Antihumanism, Metahumanism, and New Materialisms: Differences and Relations." *Existenz,* vol. 8, no. 2, pp. 26–32.

Ferrando, Francesca. 2019. *Philosophical Posthumanism.* Bloomsbury.

Flirting with Disaster. 1996. Directed by David O. Russell, Miramax.

Foundation. 2021. Created by David S. Goyer and Josh Friedman for Apple TV+. Skydance Television.

Franklin, Sarah. 2013. *Biological Relatives: IVF, Stem Cells and the Future of Kinship.* Duke UP.

Franklin, Sarah, and Susan McKinnon. 2001. *Relative Values: Reconfiguring Kinship Studies.* Duke UP.

Fuss, Diana. 1996. *Human, All Too Human.* Routledge.

Gailey, Christine Ward. 2006. "Urchins, Orphans, Monsters, and Victims: Images of Adoptive Families in U.S. Commercial Films, 1950–2000." *Adoptive Families in a Diverse Society,* edited by Katarina Wegar, Rutgers UP, pp. 71–88.

Gallagher, Catherine. 2006. "The Rise of Fictionality." *The Novel,* edited by Franco Moretti, Princeton UP, pp. 336–63.

Gledhill, Christine. 2000. "Rethinking Genre." *Reinventing Film Studies,* edited by Christine Gledhill and Linda Williams, Arnold, pp. 221–43.

Gledhill, Christine. 2018. "Prologue: The Reach of Melodrama." *Melodrama Unbound: Across History, Media, and National Cultures,* edited by Christine Gledhill and Lucinda Williams, Columbia UP, pp. ix–xxv.

Gledhill, Christine, and Linda Williams. 2018. Introduction. *Melodrama Unbound: Across History, Media, and National Cultures,* edited by Christine Gledhill and Lucinda Williams, Columbia UP, pp. 1–15.

Gleiberman, Owen. 2018. "Film Review: *Private Life.*" *Variety,* 19 Jan., https://variety.com/2018/film/reviews/private-life-review-sundance-paul-giamatti-kathryn-hahn-1202668747/.

Goldberg, Abbie E. 2019. *Open Adoptions and Diverse Families: Complex Relationships in the Digital Age.* Oxford UP.

Grant, Barry Keith. 2012. *Film Genre Reader IV.* U of Texas P.

Graves, Kori A. 2020. *A War Born Family: African American Adoption in the Wake of the Korean War.* New York UP.

Griffith, Ezra E. H., and Rachel L. Bergeron. "Cultural Stereotypes Die Hard: The Case of Transracial Adoption." *Journal of the American Academy of Psychiatry and the Law,* vol. 34, no. 3, 2006, pp. 303–314.

Grodal, Torben. 2009. *Embodied Visions: Evolution, Emotion, Culture, and Film.* Oxford UP.

The Grudge. 2004. Directed by Takashi Shimizu, Sony Pictures.

The Grudge 2. 2006. Directed by Takashi Shimizu, Sony Pictures.

The Grudge 3. 2009. Directed by Toby Wilkins, Sony Pictures.

The Grudge 4. 2020. Directed by Nicolas Pesce, Sony Pictures.

Guzikowski, Aaron. 2020a. Interview with Rachael Harper. *SciFiNow,* 9 Apr., https://www.scifinow.co.uk/tv/raised-by-wolves-interview-with-creator-aaron-guzikowski/.

Guzikowski, Aaron. 2020b. "'Raised By Wolves' Showrunner Aaron Guzikowski On Crafting An Ambitious Science Fiction World." Interview by Jack Giroux. */Film,* 7 Oct., https://www.slashfilm.com.

The Handmaid's Tale. 2017. Created by Bruce Miller, Hulu.

Haraway, Donna. 1996. "Universal Donors in Vampire Culture: It's All in the Family: Biological Kinship Categories in the Twentieth-Century United States." *Uncommon Ground: Rethinking the Human Place in Nature,* edited by William Cronon, Norton, pp. 321–78.

Haraway, Donna. 2007. "A Cyborg Manifesto: Science, Technology and Socialist-Feminism in the Late Twentieth Century." *Cybercultures Reader,* 2nd ed., edited by David Bell and Barbara M. Kennedy, Routledge, pp. 34–65. Originally published 1984.

Haraway, Donna. 2016. *Staying with the Trouble: Making Kin in the Chthulucene.* Duke UP.

Haslanger, Sally. 2009. "Family, Ancestry and Self: What Is the Moral Significance of Biological Ties?" *Adoption and Culture,* vol. 2, no. 1, pp. 91–122.

Hayles, Katherine. 2012. *How We Think: Digital Media and Contemporary Technogenesis.* U of Chicago P.

Henderson, Odie. 2019. "Luce." *Roger Ebert,* 2 Aug. https://www.rogerebert.com/reviews/luce-2019.

Hintzen, Percy, and Jean Muteba Rahier. 2014. *Problematizing Blackness: Self-Ethnographies by Black Immigrants to the United States.* Routledge.

Hipchen, Emily. 2014. "The Hyperable Adoptee: Walter Isaacson's *Steve Jobs.*" 5th Biennial International Conference on Adoption and Culture, March. Florida State University.

Hipchen, Emily. 2023. "Origins, Relinquishment, Adoption, *Frankenstein.*" Avoiding Origin Deprivation and Genetic Identity Losses: A Four-Day Symposium on Adoption and Kinship Rights, 23–26 May, School of Law, Queen's University, Belfast, Ireland.

Homans, Margaret. 2006. "Adoption Narratives, Trauma, and Origins." *Narrative,* vol. 14, no. 1, pp. 4–26.

Homans, Margaret. 2013. *The Imprint of Another Life: Adoption Narratives and Human Possibility.* U of Michigan P.

Horton, Andrew, and Johanna E. Rapf. 2013. "Comic Introduction: 'Make 'Em Laugh, Make 'Em Laugh.'" *A Companion to Film Comedy,* edited by Andrew Horton and Johanna E. Rapf, Wiley Blackwell, pp. 1–14.

Howe, Desson. 1995. Review of *Losing Isaiah. The Washington Post,* 17 Mar., https://www.washingtonpost.com/wp-srv/style/longterm/movies/videos/losingisaiahrhowe_c02a84.htm.

Hsu, Hsuan L. 2006. "Racial Privacy, the L.A. Ensemble Film, and Paul Huggis's *Crash.*" *Film Criticism,* vol. 31, no. 1, pp. 132–56.

Jacobson, Heather. 2008. *Culture Keeping: White Mothers, International Adoption, and the Negotiation of the Family Difference.* Vanderbilt UP.

Jacobson, Heather. 2014. "Framing Adoption: The Media and Parental Decision Making." *Journal of Family Issues,* vol. 35, no. 5, pp. 654–76, https://doi.org/10.1177/0192513X13479333.

Jelača, Dijana. 2018. "Alien Feminisms and Cinema's Posthuman Women." *Signs: Journal of Women in Culture and Society,* vol. 43, no. 2, pp. 379–400.

The Jerk. 1979. Directed by Michael Schultz and Carl Reiner, Universal Pictures.

Jerng, Mark. 2008. "Giving Form to Life: Cloning and Narrative Expectations of the Humans." *Partial Answers: Journal of Literature and the History of Ideas,* vol. 6, no. 2, pp. 369–93.

Jerng, Mark. 2010. *Claiming Others: Transracial Adoption and National Belonging.* U of Minnesota P.

Junior. 1994. Directed by Ivan Reitman. Universal Pictures.

Khabibullina, Lilia. 2009. "International Adoption in Russia: 'Market,' 'Children for Organs,' and 'Precious' or 'Bad' Genes." *International Adoption: Global Inequalities and the Circulation of Children,* edited by Diana Marre and Laura Briggs, New York UP, pp. 174–89.

The Kids Are Alright. 2010a. Written by Lisa Cholodenko and Stuart Blumberg. Screenplay. *IMDB,* https://www.imsdb.com/scripts/Kids-Are-All-Right,-The.html.

The Kids Are Alright. 2010b. Directed by Lisa Cholodenko, Focus Features.

Kim, Eleana. 2010. *Adopted Territory: Transnational Korean Adoptees and the Politics of Belonging.* Duke UP.

King, Geoff. 2002. *Film Comedy.* Wallflower Press.

Kline, Susan L., Amanda I. Karel, and Karishma Chatterjee. 2006. "Covering Adoption: General Depictions in Broadcast News." *Family Relations,* vol. 55, no. 4, pp. 487–98.

Kline, Susan L., Amanda I. Karel, and Karishma Chatterjee. 2009. "Healthy Depictions? Depicting Adoption and Adoption News Events on Broadcast News." *Journal of Health Communication,* vol. 14, no. 1, pp. 56–69.

Knobe, Joshua. 2011. "Finding the Mind in the Body." In *Future Science: Essays from the Cutting Edge,* edited by Max Brockman, Vintage, pp. 185–96.

Kristeva, Julia. 1992. *Powers of Horror: The Essay on Abjection.* Translated by Leon S. Roudiez, Columbia UP.

Lakoff, George, and Mark Johnson. 1980. *Metaphors We Live By.* U of Chicago P.

Lam, Carla. 2015. *New Reproductive Technologies and Disembodiment: Feminist and Material Resolutions.* Ashgate.

Latchford, Frances J. 2019. *Steeped in Blood: Adoption, Identity, and the Meaning of Family.* McGill-Queen's UP.

Latour, Bruno. 1994. "Pragmatogonies: A Mythical Account of How Humans and Nonhumans Swap Properties." *American Behavioral Scientist,* vol. 37, no. 6, pp. 791–808.

Leighton, Kimberly. 2013. "To Criticize the Right to Know We Must Question the Value of Genetic Relatedness." *American Journal of Bioethics,* vol. 13, no. 5, pp. 54–56.

Leighton, Kimberly. 2014. "Analogies to Adoption in Arguments to Anonymous Gamete Donation: Geneticizing the Desire to Know." *Family-Making: Contemporary Ethical Challenges,* edited by Francoise Baylis and Carolyn McLeod, Oxford UP, pp. 239–64.

Lévi-Strauss, Claude. 1971. *The Elementary Structures of Kinship.* Beacon Press.

Los Angeles Times Poll # 1995-360: National Issues. 1995. Conducted by *The Los Angeles Times. Roper,* https://doi.org/10.25940/ROPER-31093049.

Losing Isaiah. 1995. Directed by Stephen Gyllenhaal, Paramount.

Luce. 2019. Directed by Julius Onah, Dream Factory.

Maher, Jennifer. 2013. "Something Else Besides the Father: Reproductive Technology in Recent Hollywood Film." *Feminist Media Studies,* vol. 14, no. 5, pp. 853–67.

Mamber, Stephen. 1991. "In Search of Radical Metacinema." *Comedy/Cinema/Theory,* edited by Andrew Horton, U of California P, pp. 79–90.

Martin, Emily. 1991. "The Egg and the Sperm." *Signs,* vol 16, no. 3, pp. 485–501.

Masahiro Mori. 2012. "The Uncanny Valley." *IEEE Robotics and Automation Magazine,* vol. 19, no. 2, pp. 98–100.

Maslin, Janet. 1995. "A Little Boy and a Plot Worthy of Solomon." *New York Times,* 17 Mar., sec. C, p. 8.

McLeod, John. 2015. *Life Lines: Writing Transracial Adoption.* Bloomsbury.

McLeod, John. 2018. "Adoption and Postcolonial Inquiry." *Adoption and Culture,* vol. 6, no. 1, pp. 206–28.

McRuer, Robert. 2006. *Crip Theory: Cultural Signs of Queerness and Disability.* New York UP.

Melosh, Barbara. 2004. "Adoption Stories: Autobiographical Narrative and the Politics of Identity." *Adoption in America: Historical Perspectives,* edited by Wayne Carp, U of Michigan P, pp. 218–46.

Melosh, Barbara. 2009. *Strangers and Kin: The American Way of Adoption.* Harvard UP.

Melton, Jeffey. 2017. "Romancing the American Dream: The Coen Brothers' *Raising Arizona.*" *Studies in American Humor,* vol. 3, no. 1, pp. 1–21.

Metcalf, Greg. 2012. *The DVD Novel: How the Way We Watch Television Changed the Television We Watch.* Greenwood Publishing Group.

Mitchell, David T., and Sharon L. Snyder. 1997. Introduction. *The Body and Physical Difference: Discourses of Disability,* edited by David T. Mitchell and Sharon L. Snyder, U of Michigan P, pp. 1–35.

Modell, Judith. 2002. *A Sealed and Secret Kinship: The Culture of Policies and Practices in American Adoption.* Berghahn Books.

Mother and Child. 2010. Directed by Rodrigo Garcia, Sony Pictures Classics.

Mulhall, Stephen. 1994. "Picturing the Human (Body and Soul): A Reading of Blade Runner." *Film and Philosophy,* vol. 1, pp. 87–104.

Müller, Cornelia, and Hermann Kappelhoff. 2020. *Cinematic Metaphor: Experience, Affectivity, Temporality.* De Gruyter.

National Association of Black Social Workers. 1972. "Transracial Adoption Statement." *NABSW,* https://www.nabsw.org/sites/default/files/2024-08/NABSW_Trans-Racial_Adoption_1972_Position_%28b%29.pdf.

Nelson, Kim Park. 2006. "Shopping for Children in the International Marketplace." *Outsiders Within: Writing on Transracial Adoption,* edited by Jane Jeong Trenka et al., U of Minnesota P, pp. 89–104.

Nguyen, C. Thi, and Matthew Strohl. 2019. "Cultural Appropriation and the Intimacy of Groups." *Philosophical Studies,* vol. 176, pp. 981–1002.

Nordqvist, Petra, and Leah Gilman. 2022. *Donors: Curious Connections in Donor Conception.* Emerald Publishing.

Notini, Lauren, Christopher Gyngell, and Julian Savulescu. 2020. "Drawing the Line on In Vitro Gametogenesis." *Bioethics,* vol. 34, pp. 123–34, https://doi.org/10.1111/bioe.12679.

Novy, Marianne. 2007. *Reading Adoption: Family and Difference in Fiction and Drama.* U of Michigan P.

O'Brien, Mary. 1981. *The Politics of Reproduction.* Routledge / Kegan Paul.

O'Brien, Mary. 1989. *Reproducing the World: Essays in Feminist Theory.* Westview Press.

The Omen. 1976. Directed by Richard Donner, Mace Neufield Productions.

Orphan. 2009. Directed by Jaume Collet-Serra, Dark Castle Entertainment.

Ortiz, Ana Teresa, and Laura Briggs. 2003. "The Culture of Poverty, Crack Babies, and Welfare Cheats: The Making of the 'Healthy White Baby Crisis.'" *Social Text,* vol. 21, no. 3, pp. 39–57.

Park, Shelley M. 2013. *Mothering Queerly, Queering Motherhood: Resisting Monomaternalism in Adoptive, Lesbian, Blended, and Polygamous Families.* SUNY Press.

Patton, Sandra Lee. 2000. *Birth Marks: Transracial Adoption in Contemporary America.* New York UP.

Patton-Imani, Sandra. 2020. *Queering Family Trees: Race, Reproductive Justice, and Lesbian Motherhood.* New York UP.

Pertman, Adam. 2006. "Adoption in the Media: In Need of Editing." *Adoptive Families in a Diverse Society,* edited by Katarina Wegar, Rutgers UP, pp. 60–70.

Peters, Laura. 2000. *Orphan Texts: Victorian Orphans, Culture and Empire.* Manchester UP.

Pribram, E. Deidre. 2018. "Melodrama and the Aesthetic of Emotion." *Melodrama Unbound: Across History, Media, and National Cultures,* edited by Christine Gledhill and Lucinda Williams, Columbia UP, pp. 237–52.

Prince, Stephen. 2004. *The Horror Film.* Rutgers UP.

Private Life. 2018. Directed by Tamara Jenkins. Netflix.

Raised by Wolves. 2020. Created by Aaron Guzikowski, HBO Max. Scott Free Productions.

Raising Arizona. 1987. Directed by Ethan Coen and Joel Coen, 20th Century Fox.

Renner, Karen J. 2013. "Evil Children in Film and Literature." *The "Evil Child" in Literature, Film, and Popular Culture,* edited by Karen J. Renner, Routledge, pp. 1–27.

"Reproductive Techno-Horror Is a Burgeoning Genre on Screen." 2023. *The Economist,* 2 May, https://www.economist.com/culture/2023/05/02/reproductive-techno-horror-is-a-burgeoning-genre-on-screen.

The Ring. 2002. Directed by Gore Verbinski, DreamWorks Pictures.

Roberts, Dorothy. 2022. *Torn Apart: How the Child Welfare System Destroys Black Families—And How Abolition Can Build a Safer World.* Basic Books.

Robinson, Katy. 2002. *A Single Square Picture.* Berkley Books.

Rudy, Sayres. 2019. "The Anxious Kinship of the Vanishing Adoptee." *Adoption and Culture,* vol. 7, no. 2, The Ohio State UP, pp. 206–29.

Russell, David O. 1996. *"Flirting with Disaster," and "Spanking the Monkey."* Screenplay. Boston: Faber and Faber.

Sales, Sally. 2012. *Adoption, Family, and the Paradox of Origins: A Foucauldian History.* Palgrave Macmillan.

Sanders, Joe. 1994. "*Raising Arizona*: Not-Quite Ozzie and Harriet Meet the Biker from Hell." *The Doppelgänger in Contemporary Literature, Film, and Art,* double special issue of *Journal of the Fantastic in the Arts,* vol. 6, nos. 2–3 (22–23), pp. 217–33.

Scahill, Andrew. 2015. *The Revolting Child in Horror Cinema: Youth Rebellion and Queer Spectatorship.* Palgrave Macmillan.

Shanahan, Timothy, and Paul Smart. 2020. *Blade Runner 2049: A Philosophical Exploration.* Routledge.

Sharma, Devika, and Frederik Tygstrup. 2015. *Structures of Feeling: Affectivity and the Study of Culture.* De Gruyter.

Shildrick, Margrit. 2002. *Embodying the Monster: Encounters with the Vulnerable Self.* Sage.

Siebers, Tobin. 2008. *Disability Theory.* U of Michigan P.

Silent Hill. 2006. Directed by Christophe Gans and M. J. Bassett, Konami.

Silvey, Vivien. 2013. "Pluralism and Cultural Imperialism in the Network Films *Babel* and *Lantana.*" *Journal of Postcolonial Writing,* vol. 49, no. 5, pp. 582–95, https://doi.org/10.1080/17449855.2013.842738.

Singley, Carol J. 2011. *Adopting America: Childhood, Kinship, and National Identity in Literature.* Oxford UP.

Smolin, David. 2012. "Of Orphans and Adoption, Parents and the Poor, Exploitation and Rescue: A Scriptural and Theological Critique of the Evangelical Christian Adoption and Orphan Care Movement." *Regent Journal of International Law,* vol 8., no. 2, pp. 267–24.

Splice. 2009. Directed by Vincenzo Natali, Warner Bros.

Squier, Susan Merrill. 2004. *Liminal Lives: Imagining the Human at the Frontiers of Biomedicine*. Duke UP.

Stewart, Will. 2010. "Fury as U.S. Woman Adopts Russian Boy, 7, Then Sends Him Back Alone with Note Saying: 'I Don't Want Him Anymore.'" *Daily Mail*, 10 Apr., https://www.dailymail.co.uk/news/article-1264744/American-sends-adopted-Russian-boy-behavioural-problems.html.

Strathern, Marilyn. 1992. *Reproducing the Future: Anthropology, Kinship, and New Reproductive Technologies*. Routledge / Chapman and Hall.

Trenka, Jane Jeong. 2003. *The Language of Blood*. Borealis Books.

"2020 Survey." 2023. *We Are Donor Conceived*, 22 Sept., https://www.wearedonorconceived.com/2020-we-are-donor-conceived-survey/.

van der Ploeg, Irma. 2001. *Prosthetic Bodies: The Construction of the Fetus and the Couple as Patients in Reproductive Technologies*. Kluwer Academic.

Vint, Sherryl. 2021. *Science Fiction*. MIT Press.

Wegar, Katarina. 1997. *Adoption, Identity, and Fiction: The Debate over Sealed Birth Records*. Yale UP.

Weitz, Eric. 2009. *The Cambridge Introduction to Comedy*. Cambridge UP.

Wiggins, Daphne Nell. 1996. "The Multiethnic Placement Act of 1994: Background, Purpose, Interpretations and Effects of Legislation Regarding Transracial Adoption." *Law and Psychology Review*, vol. 20, pp. 275–90.

Williams Raymond. 2009. "On Structure of Feeling." *Emotions: A Cultural Studies Reader*, edited by Jennifer Harding and E. Deidre Pribram, Routledge, pp. 35–49.

Williams, Raymond, and Michael Orrom. 1954. *Preface to Film*. Film Drama Limited.

Winslow, Rachel Rains. 2017. *The Best Possible Immigrants: International Adoption and the American Family*. U of Pennsylvania P.

Witt, Charlotte. 2014. "A Critique of the Bionormative Concept of the Family." *Family-Making: Contemporary Ethical Challenges*, edited by Francoise Baylis and Carolyn McLeod, Oxford UP, pp. 49–63.

Zelizer, Viviana. 1985. *Pricing the Priceless Child: The Changing Social Value of Children*. Basic.

Ziff, Bruce H., and Pratima V. Rao. 1997. *Borrowed Power: Essays on Cultural Appropriation*. Rutgers UP.

INDEX

FORMATIONS: ADOPTION, KINSHIP, AND CULTURE

EMILY HIPCHEN AND JOHN McLEOD, SERIES EDITORS

This interdisciplinary series encourages critical engagement with all aspects of nonnormative kinship—such as adoption, foster care, IVF, surrogacy, and gamete transfers—especially as they intersect with race, identity, heritage, nationality, sexuality, and gender. Books in the series explore how these constructions affect not only those personally involved but also public understandings of identity, personhood, migration, kinship, and the politics of family.

Kinflix: Adoption and Assisted Reproductive Technologies in Film
Marina Fedosik

Unsettling Acts: Performing Transnational Adoption
Jieun Lee

Haphazard Families: Romanticism, Nation, and the Prehistory of Modern Adoption
Eric C. Walker

Adoption Fantasies: The Fetishization of Asian Adoptees from Girlhood to Womanhood
Kimberly D. McKee

Adoption across Race and Nation: US Histories and Legacies
Edited by Silke Hackenesch

The Politics of Reproduction: Adoption, Abortion, and Surrogacy in the Age of Neoliberalism
Edited by Modhumita Roy and Mary Thompson

"Books on God's existence have, of course, been written. But rarely have they been written by such a thoughtful and erudite collection of individuals, as is the case in this book. The volume is a great resource for both introducing and thoroughly engaging with some of the most important arguments surrounding the question of God's existence. With entries from both believers and nonbelievers, the book aims to help you figure out for yourself how to think about the question."

—**Alex O'Connor,** host of the podcast *Within Reason*

"*Debating God's Existence* is my new go-to book for believers and skeptics who want to understand the arguments for and against God. Both the tone and content of the dialogue are first-rate. Authors cover the big issues at the center of the debate about God's existence—the origin and fine-tuning of the universe, morality, and the hiddenness of God. This book strikes a rare balance of being understandable for nonexperts while offering fresh insights for scholars."

—**Sean McDowell,** associate professor of Christian apologetics,
Talbot School of Theology

"This book feels like sitting at the table with deep thinkers on both sides of the God question—and actually getting somewhere. The book doesn't try to force conclusions but invites readers to think more clearly, listen more charitably, and disagree more honestly. It's thoughtful without being stuffy, deep without being preachy, and respectful without pulling punches. I recommend it to anyone who wants more light than heat in these conversations."

—**Michael Licona,** professor of New Testament Studies, Houston Christian University

"Too often discussions between theists and nontheists assume a competitive, 'I win, you lose' mentality. How might truth be better served if disagreements about God were conducted with more respect for the other side—even, as appropriate, more empathy and compassion? This fascinating book models a better way forward, not only containing contributions from both theists and nontheists but involving some of the leading and most influential philosophers of religion of our time. In sum, this book is an invaluable resource for anyone engaged in conversation about the existence of God."

—**Gavin Ortlund,** president of Truth Unites;
theologian in residence at Immanuel Nashville

"This book is a unique resource for anyone struggling with (or merely wondering about) the reality of a divine creator. Almost every known argument is put forward and subjected to criticism from the other side. As Paul Copan says in his preface, these criticisms are far from the useless harangues one sees on internet debates; instead, they are scholarly, respectful, and worthy of consideration. In our increasingly bitter and divisive culture where civilized debates have become rare, this book stands as a model for how we might return to a more harmonious, loving, and Christ-centered way of thinking, discussing, and living."

—**Sy Garte,** former director of physiological and pathological sciences,
NIH Center for Scientific Review

"Civilized debate aimed at truth and mutual understanding is a rarity today. How refreshing, then, is this carefully curated, robust yet respectful interchange between leading proponents of atheism and theism! The format provides a level playing field for exploring the great questions of God's existence, the problem of evil, divine hiddenness, fine-tuning, the foundation of morality, and the possibility of immaterial beings. Readers will gain both greater understanding of the issues and greater respect for those with whom they disagree."

—**Angus J. L. Menuge,** professor of philosophy, Concordia University of Wisconsin; past president of the Evangelical Philosophical Society

"This book brings together a diverse range of thinkers to debate the existence of God. Senior and junior scholars, philosophers of science, ethicists, and more are brought into an engaging conversation over one of life's biggest questions. Readers will learn a great deal from this insightful exchange."

—**R. T. Mullins,** lecturer and researcher in philosophy, theology, and religions, University of Lucerne

"Healthy debate is important. Healthy debate about God is of supreme importance. Whether you believe that God exists or not, this book will challenge, inspire, frustrate, press, and hopefully help you come to your own conclusion about ultimate reality. Don't let the friendly tone of the initial debate between Johnson and Barker fool you: Sophisticated arguments and counterarguments about God's existence and nature, as the extended discussions in this volume reveal, demand our sustained attention. Read the book, follow the arguments, weigh the evidence, and consider afresh the question of God."

—**Paul M. Gould,** professor of philosophy of religion, director of the Master of Arts in philosophy of religion program, Palm Beach Atlantic University

"The most striking thing to me about this collection of essays is the impressive lineup of Christian theists writing in support of God's existence. Truly, as a result of the renaissance of Christian philosophy over the last generation, Christian thinkers no longer find themselves beleaguered and on the defensive, but quite the contrary, are now better equipped to make their case than their opponents."

—**William Lane Craig,** Emeritus Research Professor of Philosophy, Talbot School of Theology

"The response essays provide an accessible but cutting-edge introduction to some of the most important points of contact between theism and atheism. Well worth a read."

—**Luke Barnes,** astrophysicist and lecturer, Western Sydney University

"*Debating God's Existence* is a superb example of atheists and theists seeking to collaborate in pursuit of truth. I highly recommend this book; it's a model of collaboration on an all-important topic with implications for us all."

—**Corey Miller,** president of Ratio Christi

"*Debating God's Existence* is a must read for anyone interested in contemporary philosophy of religion—especially those engaging its central question: Does God exist? Drinkard has assembled an all-star cast of contributors who argue their respective positions with clarity and rigor. The book accomplishes a rare feat: It functions equally well as a college textbook and a truly novel contribution to the field."

—**Michael DeVito,** lecturer in philosophy, University of Maine; former NFL player for the New York Jets and Kansas City Chiefs